OGIER'S
READING
RESEARCH

How to make research
more approachable

THIRD EDITION

Edited by

Nicky Lanoë

RGN, RCNT, RNT, MSc, ILTM
Freelance Lecturer/Consultant
St Martins, Guernsey, Channel Islands

Foreword by

Margaret E Ogier

RGN, RM, DipN, RNT, BSc, PhD, C Psychol
Freelance Lecturer/Researcher
Castel, Guernsey, Channel Islands

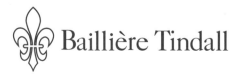

Baillière Tindall

EDINBURGH LONDON NEW YORK OXFORD PHILADELPHIA ST LOUIS SYDNEY
TORONTO 1991

BAILLIÈRE TINDALL
An imprint of Elsevier Limited

First published 1989
Second editon 1998
Third edition 2002
    Reprinted 2003, 2004, 2005, 2006, 2007

ISBN-13: 978–0–7020–2670–6
ISBN-10: 0–7020–2670–0

British Library Cataloguing in Publication Data
A catalogue record for this book is available from the British Library

Library of Congress Cataloging in Publication Data
A catalog record for this book is available from the Library of Congress

Note
Medical knowledge is constantly changing. As new information becomes
available, changes in treatment, procedures, equipment and the use of
drugs become necessary. The editors, contributor and the publishers have
taken care to ensure that the information given in this text is accurate and
up to date. However, readers are strongly advised to confirm that the
information, especially with regard to drug usage, complies with the latest
legislation and standards of practice.

The Publisher

Key words:
- Understanding research
- Evidence-based practice
- Information technology
- Nursing
- Literature search

your source for books,
journals and multimedia
in the health sciences

www.elsevierhealth.com

Working together to grow
libraries in developing countries

www.elsevier.com | www.bookaid.org | www.sabre.org

ELSEVIER   BOOK AID International   Sabre Foundation

The
publisher's
policy is to use
paper manufactured
from sustainable forests

Printed in China
B/06

OGIER'S READING RESEARCH

How to make research more approachable

For Baillière Tindall

Senior Commissioning Editor: Sarena Wolfaard
Project Development Manager: Karen Gilmour
Project Manager: Joannah Duncan
Design Direction: Judith Wright

Contents

Foreword

In the last thirteen years since the first edition of *Reading Research* was published, nurses are better informed about nursing practice related to research findings. However, the word research still produces shivers of horror for neophyte and some experienced nurses. In addition, over the intervening thirteen years since the first edition, information technology has made enormous advances and provided rapid, easy access to vast amounts of information, research, data, opinions and facts. Whilst its ready source of knowledge is welcomed, it brings with it issues of discernment and learning such as the identification of reliable and valid research data, as opposed to informed opinion.

It is, therefore, with pleasure that I recommend to you Nicky Lanoë's updating of *Reading Research*. Nicky has brought to this third edition her wide experience as a nurse lecturer and researcher, ably dealing with both the issues of professional practice and the understanding of research in the context of two rapidly changing fields of expertise.

The essential essence of *Reading Research* as a text is to get you started in finding, then reading with understanding, research. This has been maintained in this new edition, whilst updating the material to equip the nurse of the 21st century and onwards with the basic research knowledge to be a safe practitioner for the safety of the patient/client, and to meet their own professional requirement and integrity.

Margaret Ogier 2002

Acknowledgements

Acknowledgements to the second edition

Thanks are due to many people who have contributed their knowledge, expertise and enthusiasm at various points from the inception to publication of this booklet:

Without the good will and hard work of many trained nurses, from enrolled to senior nurse managers and educators, who have attended the Research Workshops upon which this booklet is based, the ideas and concepts would not have evolved.

To Caroline Foster-Doan, the late Harry Gallagher, Heather Gough, and Pierre Herve thanks for reading the preliminary manuscript, commenting and encouraging me to offer the booklet for publication.

To the nurse researchers who reviewed the manuscript and gave of their time and expertise to refine and improve the original concepts, I owe a large debt of gratitude.

For the clarity of expression, enthusiasm and support I sincerely thank Richenda Milton-Thompson. My thanks go, too, to Michael Dixon for advice on the Results section.

If it had not been for Rosemary Morris, Carrie Walker and the staff at Scutari publishers showing patience and faith in this booklet it would not have reached this stage. To you all many thanks.

Many thanks to you the nurses who have read and used the first edition and encouraged the writing of a second edition.

I appreciate the advice and expertise of the reviewers and nurse researchers who have willingly shared their work.

Without the help of several librarians such as those at the Royal College of Nursing and Valerie Rowland and Ruth Smale of the Nurse Education Library, Guernsey, who with patience and good humour found the most obscure journal articles and followed up references for me, writing this second edition would have been impossible.

Thanks to Jacqui Curthoys of Baillière Tindall for her support, enthusiasm and bright ideas.

Special thanks to my husband John for his support in many different ways and his patience while I disappeared under piles of paper and books.

Without the efforts of all mentioned above the material would not have appeared in the form it is today. While every effort has been taken to be accurate while being brief, as author, I accept the responsibility for any weakness or inaccuracy.

Margaret Ogier

Acknowledgements for the third edition

Over and above Margaret's supporters, especially Val, who has yet again provided me with an impeccable service, I would like to take this opportunity to thank the following:

First, I would like to thank Margaret herself. I know that of all the many books she has written this was in many ways her best loved. Hence it was a great honour to be asked to edit this edition, and one I did not undertake lightly. Margaret has been my long-term mentor, colleague and dear friend. I hope I have managed to keep to the spirit of the book while updating it in line with current developments.

Second, I would like to thank all the reviewers for their useful and constructive feedback. In particular I would like to thank my sister, Jane Rushton, who works as a practice nurse, and Ann Martin, formerly my degree student and now Director of Nursing at our local hospice. Both came to studying research for the first time later on in their careers and their insights were most helpful.

Nicky Lanoë

1

Introduction: how to use this book

Key words:
- Informed practice
- Evidence-based practice
- Research-based profession

> Research? That's something people do in university departments or laboratories isn't it? It doesn't have much to do with real life does it? Isn't it something nurses do if they feel they are not very good at proper hands on care?

This is the opening remark from the first edition of this book, written in 1989. For a few readers the sentiments might still be true, but many more nurses now are aware of the key role of research, or at least acknowledge the importance of research findings in informed practice. This is a natural and desired consequence of the evolution of pre- and post-registration education, and indeed the evolution of nursing as a profession in its own right.

However, there is still a substantial population of nurses (and indeed other healthcare practitioners) who, for a variety of reasons, feel ill-equipped to find, read and critically evaluate research. Perhaps you are embarking on a health-related BTec or Access course with a view to a career in nursing or an allied profession. Alternatively, you might just be starting out on your nursing career and want to gain an overview of your role in relation to research. Possibly you wish to prepare for some post-registration initiative, like a Level 3 course. Perhaps, like me, you qualified a long time ago and feel the need to update your skills, or have had a career break and plan to undertake a back-to-nursing course. Or perhaps, like so many colleagues I have met over the years, you have for some reason just been frightened off research. If any of these apply, then this book is for you!

Thus, this third edition retains the original aim from the first edition: to make reading research reports a feasible and enjoyable task. If you can find a way of interpreting and understanding research then you will be working towards **evidence-based practice**. You should develop an awareness of research findings together with critical reading skills so that you can be selective in choosing the most appropriate findings and, where necessary, seek further support for some findings and discard others on an informed basis. With the drive to make nursing a **research-based profession** there is a danger that, rather than rejecting research, as in the opening quotation, nurses might feel compelled to adopt a particular piece of research just because it *is* research, without giving the results and their implications due critical, knowledgeable scrutiny.

This book is intended as a guide to help you avoid these pitfalls, and also as a stimulus for further reading and appreciation of nursing research. It is written from experience of working with qualified nurses who have not encountered research reports previously. It is not intended to belittle what you already know, but rather to build on your current knowledge, skills and, importantly, engender a positive attitude towards research.

As the text is designed to be readable and concise (it is purposefully kept small to fit in your pocket), it is inevitable that some terms, ideas and issues will not be mentioned or explored fully. Many detailed books are available on aspects of the research process, some more readable than others. This book does not aim to compete with these, but rather gives you a 'jumping-off point' from which to tackle them. When you read Chapter 3 about how to find what you need to read, it would be useful to check what other research texts are available in your local library or resource centre to complement this text. For example, the work by Burns & Grove (2001) is a useful resource. This American text presents a more detailed exploration of quantitative and qualitative methodologies and also investigates best practices and evidence-based practice. There are, however, many others available from a vast range of geographical perspectives – find out what is available in your area to meet your needs.

Above all, this text does not prepare you to do research. Indeed, Mead (1996) highlights the dangers of students and nurses attempting small-scale research projects as part of their educational programme. In my own experience, I did not feel equipped with the knowledge or skills to undertake research until studying for my Master's degree, and then with close supervision. This, however, in no way negates the important role you have to play in the research process.

How to use this book

The key words at the start of this introductory chapter gave a hint of the main topics included in the chapter. Each chapter contains key words that are in bold type in the text.

Icons in the margin indicate where there is further reading (📖), reference to a term in the Glossary (**G** ⮞) or a cross-reference.

In order to help explain a point, brief boxed examples are included.

Short self-assessment questions are included at various points and are indicated by 📖 in the margin. Do undertake these, however tempting it might seem to gloss over them. It helps to make your learning an active process, rather than just passively reading the text. It also helps you to consider issues in the light of your practice – an important consideration.

To this end too, if you own this text, do make use of the margins to jot down your own feelings and thoughts, underline key points, highlight issues for further exploration, and so on. Obviously, if you are using a library copy this is not possible, so you might find it useful to make separate notes.

The next chapter considers the reasons for doing research. Chapter 3 discusses how to find research reports. After that, each chapter follows the order of a research report, addressing each section in turn, i.e. literature review, method, results, and so on.

2

Why bother about research?

Key words:
- Clinical governance
- Clinical effectiveness
- Nursing excellence
- Knowledge

The first thorny question to address must be: why bother about nursing research at all? As you are already reading this book, perhaps you are clear as to why this is important. However, we all need motivating from time to time and reviewing the purpose of any activity helps to achieve this goal. This chapter therefore briefly considers political, professional, clinical and personal reasons why the understanding and application of nursing research findings are important.

Political influences

Historically in nursing, change tended to be imposed from 'the top down'. Edicts were generated by the government and the higher echelons of the profession and 'imposed' in many ways on those in practice. Such top-down approaches when trying to foster change at least partially explain why nurses at the grass roots were slow to, or rejected attempts to, develop their research-based practice. For example, The Report of the Committee on Nursing (Briggs Report) (Department of Health and Social Security et al, 1972) stressed the need for nursing courses and hence practices to incorporate research methods and their critical usage. However, in reality, very little altered over the next 20 years.

Times move on though and, for a variety of reasons, the impetus and approach behind such initiatives have changed. For example, it is now more overtly recognised that nurses are expensive resources and must therefore be able to demonstrate their worth through the identification of research- and evidence-based outcomes of care. Strategies for nursing at national, regional and local levels therefore need to reflect a real commitment to such practice both in terms of value for money and quality of patient care.

The philosophy (reasoned way of thinking) that underpins the 'new' National Health Service (NHS) is reflected in a variety of reports (Department of Health, 1993a, 1994, 1996, 1997, 1998, Moores 1996). Two important initiatives that have evolved from a combination of such philosophies are **clinical governance** and **clinical effectiveness**.

Clinical governance is not a new concept in itself, rather, it is an amalgamation of a range of components such as evidence-based practice; policy audit, evaluation, accountability and performance; the meaningful involvement of patients and the public; and so on. It highlights the importance of making quality everyone's business. Whereas this at present relates directly to the NHS, the underlying principles are, or should be, easily applied to any healthcare setting.

At face value this could seem to be an organisational responsibility. However, a United Kingdom Central Council for Nursing, Midwifery and Health Visiting Publication entitled *Professional self-regulation and clinical governance* (UKCC 2001a) provides a useful review of the role of the individual practitioner in relation to clinical governance. In essence, this publication reminds practitioners that clinical governance requires them to promote good, and prevent poor, practice, and (importantly) to intervene in unacceptable practice. This strengthens the need for all practitioners to be accountable for their care and to maintain and promote high standards of patient/client care.

Clinical effectiveness, therefore, is one vital element of clinical governance. Being clinically effective can be simplistically defined as 'doing the right thing' rather than just merely 'doing things right'. It is about being able to demonstrate that nursing interventions do what they set out to do to maintain and improve health, within the available resources. This, again, strengthens the case for every practitioner to base his or her care on the best possible evidence. To explore these issues further, a useful resource is the book by Chambers & Boath (2001). In addition, the work by the Foundation of Nursing Studies (2000) is of value.

Professional development

Perhaps a good place to start is with a quotation:

> When nurses' sensitivity to human needs (their intuition) is joined with the ability to find and use expert opinion, with the ability to find reported research and apply it to their practice, and when they themselves use the scientific method of investigation, there is no limit to the influence they might have on health care worldwide. (Henderson 1987)

This sentiment, I am sure, is one with which the majority of nurses would concur. This **excellence** and commitment demanded of nurses is reinforced by the UKCC (1992) Code of Professional Conduct (and is maintained in the new edition to be published in 2002), which exhorts all nurses, midwives and health visitors to:

> Act always in such a manner as to promote and safeguard the interest and well-being of patients and clients ... [and] maintain and improve your professional knowledge and competence.

Nurses who are content to learn by rote and continue to perform a particular procedure because 'it has always been done that way' in their area of practice will never approach this level of excellence. Indeed, the care they deliver could be actually harmful and bad, however well intended.

The Code of Conduct is further reinforced by the UKCC's PREP initiative (UKCC 2001b). These standards require all nurses to keep up to date with new developments in practice, to think and reflect for themselves and to demonstrate the same by providing the best possible care for their clients. It is the responsibility of all practitioners to document evidence of these achievements and to state that they have fulfilled them when re-registering. To maintain quality, a sample of nurses is audited and asked to provide a synopsis of such evidence.

Clinical development

One area of practice of importance to many nurses and in which the value of research findings can be easily seen is in the care of pressure areas. There has been an enormous amount of research conducted on this topic since the pioneering work of Doreen Norton in 1962 (Norton et al 1962). Indeed, there are recently published evidence-based guidelines (Royal College of

Nursing 2001) on pressure ulcer risk assessment and prevention. Unfortunately, however, there are still wards and hospitals throughout the country where research is considered to
be something that has no relation to clinical nursing, and
harmful practices remain in use. Indeed, ideas on treatments
are sometimes as varied as the individual nurses. Many rituals
persist, even though they have been shown to be harmful. A
good, if frightening read is the book by Ford & Walsh (1994),
which explores just such issues.

see
Chapter 3

Carrying out a computer-based literature search (using
CINAHL) to update the references for this edition, I found
464 journal articles in 2001 related to pressure areas and the
variety of methods to relieve pressure (there were only 18 in
1995 – an interesting point to note). So there is plenty of
research going on and it is being reported in accessible journals
held in most local libraries. However, it is doubtful that research
findings are being widely used to inform everyday practice.

As indicated in the report *Strategy for research in nursing,
midwifery and health visiting* (Department of Health 1993b,
Annexe 3.2.3):

> There is a need to create a climate where research is respected and
> used in practice. Managers, practitioners and educators should all
> be a part of this process. There is also a clear role for both pur-
> chaser and providers.

Another important area to consider is the psychological
aspect of care. How much do we depersonalise patients and
staff? In Ogier's (1982) work, student nurses felt happier and
thought they had learned more in wards where other staff
recognised them as individuals – as Mary or David – and
not just another student. More recent work (Amos 2001),
examining the transition of students to the role of Staff Nurse,
supports this. Friendliness and approachability of preceptors
was deemed an important issue in terms of helpful support.
The ability to address another person by name does not
require a complex educational programme; rather it is a basic
courtesy that research has shown to be missing in many
instances. By increased sensitivity to the needs of others,
patient care and staff morale can be inexpensively improved.
This is not to say that training in communication and interpersonal skills should not be given. Indeed, the need for these was

highlighted many years ago by several researchers (e.g. Gott 1984, Powell 1982).

One community health council carried out a year-long survey to monitor the quality of information-giving, with a sample of 1500 patients discharged from acute hospitals. The results show a generally high level of satisfaction with the information related to surgical and technical procedures. Less technical aspects of care, such as reasons for bed rest, were less well explained. Some patients found staff insensitive in the way that they conveyed upsetting or disappointing news (Cortis & Lacey 1996). A nurse colleague of mine who has recently been hospitalised supported this, especially in relation to psychological care. He stated that domestic workers provided the most effective 'caring'. This anecdotal evidence could perhaps benefit from being researched in its own right. For example, it could perhaps be a reflection of a broader issue: are there particular issues we need to consider when caring for colleagues?

At a deeper level of interpersonal understanding, Twomey (1987) suggests that we should look more closely at what patients actually need, and not jump to conclusions as to what we think they need. In considering Ann Tait's in-depth study of one patient, Twomey looks at the issues surrounding the woman who undergoes a mastectomy. She identifies the concerns of many women as being not only with the mutilation but also with the implications of having cancer. Faulkner (1984), amongst others, looked at the incidence of clinical depression in women who had mastectomies and the role of the nurse in helping patients adjust to the trauma. In an effort to compensate for some of these weaknesses, Edmonstone (1996) reports on an initiative by the Scottish Department of Health to carry out a research programme that would empower nurses working with cancer patients. If these issues concern you in particular, or relate specifically to your area of practice, why not seek out and read the original research studies.

All this might sound very academic but just think for a moment. If someone close to you had just undergone a traumatic operation, you would want every opportunity to be taken to help him or her adjust to a new body image without further distress. If you think about it as a caring nurse rather than as a concerned relative, you would probably wish the same. As a nurse, familiarity with research findings in a number of studies, including those cited here, will make it easier for you to achieve this.

Personal development

As noted earlier, research studies look at nursing and nurses as well as patients. For instance, research into the influences on nursing staff's perception of stress in the operating theatre has shown that difficulties with the organisation of staff meal breaks produces highly significant stress levels (Astbury 1988). Spouse (1990) highlights the stress on both the qualified nurse and the student as they try to match service and educational needs within the clinical area.

'Knowledge is power' is a very old saying. What familiarity with research findings does is to broaden your **knowledge** and give you ammunition to use in your fight for better care, better opportunities and better quality of life for your patients. Familiarity with research findings can help you to avoid complications that are costly in terms of money and human suffering. Such familiarity could also broaden your knowledge in such a way as to enable you to make conditions better and learning easier for you and your colleagues. The secret lies in knowing how to access research findings, to evaluate research reports and how to implement appropriate findings, thereby beginning to bridge the theory–practice gap. It also alerts you as to areas where more research is necessary. To reiterate, this is *not* to mean that it is your responsibility to undertake the research, but certainly all nurses are in a position where they need to raise such areas of concern. This could be to colleagues whose remit includes such research activities, or to the wider profession through letters to nursing journals.

Have a break now and reflect on what you have been reading. Are you now clear as to what the political, professional, clinical and personal reasons are for needing to be able to understand and apply nursing research? Are there any others that you personally would like to add?

The next chapter moves on from the why to the how: having determined a problem you wish to explore, how do you go about finding relevant and credible research?

3

How to find what you need to read

Key words:
- Key words
- Synonyms
- Information technology
  - *Database*
  - *MEDLINE*
  - *CINAHL*
  - *BNI*
  - *Cochrane Library*
  - *Internet/website*
- Abstracting journals

If you have found a research report you want to read, or if you have been given a piece of research to study, then you are ready to start. If not, you might like to 'browse' through some journals and identify research reports to whet your appetite.

There is a multitude of nursing journals so it can be difficult to know where to start. In the Further Reading section, I have indicated some that contain more research reports than others. Breed (1999), for example, offers a useful review of 40 health-care journals. Stodulski (1995) too carried out a study of UK nursing journals and rated the journals for levels of research content; the following are those rated as containing high levels of research:

- *Intensive and Critical Care Nursing*
- *International Journal of Nursing Studies*
- *Journal of Advanced Nursing*
- *Midwifery*
- *Nurse Education Today*
- *Nurse Researcher.*

I would also add to this list the more recently published international journal *Evidence-Based Nursing*. These might be a starting point to identify a journal with high research content if you just want to familiarise yourself with the type of relevant article. Obviously your particular interests, geographical location and area of practice will ultimately guide your choice.

It is important to note that more and more journals are now increasing their research content as the drive for evidence-based practice and a research-based profession continues. This is reflected in the way they accept articles for publication. A 'blind review' is undertaken by peers who are not told the names(s) of the researcher(s), nor is the researcher(s) told the names of the reviewers. This is always highlighted in the fly-sheet of the journals and is useful to check as it is one indication of 'quality'.

Starting point

First, clarify the topic. For example, if you have not been given a particular issue to investigate for a course assignment, but there is a particular question you would like to investigate, the first step is to write it out in your own words.

> The question Ogier (1982) wanted to answer when she had the opportunity to carry out some research was: 'What is it about some ward sisters that they make student nurses feel they have learnt something, while with other sisters, students are left with the feeling that they have just survived an obstacle course?' (I know this book is not about you carrying out research but the starting point is the same. To research into anything, you have to find out what is already known; in other words you have to carry out a literature search to look for research studies already carried out in that area and identify any gaps.)

You might consider Ogier's (1982) work, albeit seminal, to be rather dated and indeed it is always wise to be cautious when reading research of such an age. It can be useful when searching the literature to set a time span of, say, up to 5 years. Conversely, should you find quality research of interest that is older than this, then it is useful to determine whether it has been replicated or what else has been undertaken in a similar area. For example, recent work undertaken by Evans (2001) explored the expectations of newly qualified nurses and the methodology and findings closely mirrored Ogier's (1982), even though the nature of the participants was different.

It is useful to share and discuss your ideas with colleagues and friends. Rethink your question in the light of the discussions that arise from sharing it. It is wise to do this on several occasions, as each time you explain your ideas you are clarifying and refining them. It can be particularly helpful to find a non-nurse willing to listen to your ideas. A layperson is likely to question aspects that we as nurses take for granted or as unchallenged facts.

Now you might need, or like, to rewrite your original idea. Ogier's (1982) final research question was: 'What is it about a ward sister's leadership style and verbal interaction with nurse learners that affects their (the student's) learning?' (The term 'Sister' now appears rather sexist and dated, having been in the main replaced with Charge Nurse or the equivalent, depending on the geographical location of the post-holder.)

Next, underline the **key words** (to be manageable, there should be no more than six of these). From the example above, the key words might be 'sister' and 'learning'.

List the key words and beside each write as many **synonyms** or words that you think mean the same or are closely similar:

- Sister: charge nurse, head nurse
- Learning: studying, teaching, understanding.

What is the point of this exercise? If you are like me, you are no doubt short of time and rush into the library 15 minutes before it is due to close. By the time you have caught your breath and decided what it is you want, you are being asked to leave. However, if you have spent some time thinking through your ideas before you rush into the library, you will be able to make a coherent request to the librarian, who will be much better able to help you. Or, if you make your own search, you will at least know where to start. I suggest you put alternatives next to your key words because your first word might draw a blank in the subject index. 'Sister' is not likely to draw a blank, but you are in danger of being overwhelmed with information. However, if you search for 'kidneys' you might not get many references, but by using the words 'renal' or 'urology' you will soon find relevant articles.

BAILLIÈRE TINDALL
An imprint of Elsevier Limited

First published 1989
Second editon 1998
Third edition 2002
   Reprinted 2003, 2004, 2005, 2006, 2007

ISBN-13: 978–0–7020–2670–6
ISBN-10: 0–7020–2670–0

British Library Cataloguing in Publication Data
A catalogue record for this book is available from the British Library

Library of Congress Cataloging in Publication Data
A catalog record for this book is available from the Library of Congress

Note
Medical knowledge is constantly changing. As new information becomes available, changes in treatment, procedures, equipment and the use of drugs become necessary. The editors, contributor and the publishers have taken care to ensure that the information given in this text is accurate and up to date. However, readers are strongly advised to confirm that the information, especially with regard to drug usage, complies with the latest legislation and standards of practice.

The Publisher

Key words:
- Understanding research
- Evidence-based practice
- Information technology
- Nursing
- Literature search

ELSEVIER
your source for books,
journals and multimedia
in the health sciences
www.elsevierhealth.com

Working together to grow
libraries in developing countries

www.elsevier.com | www.bookaid.org | www.sabre.org

ELSEVIER   BOOK AID International   Sabre Foundation

The publisher's policy is to use paper manufactured from sustainable forests

Printed in China
B/06

Figure 3.1   Sample bibliographic page.

Key words and their synonyms help you find relevant material. When you have identified something interesting, key words are useful again: if you turn to the back of the title page in most published books and reports you will find a list of key words provided by the author for the British Library Cataloguing in Publication Data (Fig. 3.1). Compare your list with the author's to get an idea of whether the text will be useful to you.

Getting help from information technology

Information technology has revolutionised the next part of the literature search and can save a lot of time and energy. When preparing material for this edition, 2 hours spent at a computer terminal in the local library generated as many references as I would have gathered in 2 weeks manually searching indexes and abstracting journals. Do not be intimidated by the mention of technology; most libraries will provide the novice with an instruction sheet as to which buttons to push and when and where to type in the key words. Below are a few terms you may hear used in connection with computer-generated searches.

Data (datum singular) are information or facts. Therefore, a **database** is a source that contains information or facts, rather like a telephone directory, but in this case, author names, titles of journals and books with a brief summary, and date of publication. The database could be a fact file, but more frequently refers to computer storage. Computerisation enables searches to be made quickly because links between entries and various combinations can be identified (see the example below on stab wounds of the chest).

CD-ROM (compact disk read-only memory) is a means of storing relevant information that cannot be altered, e.g. titles, authors and summaries of research reports, journal articles or books. The disk is inserted into the computer and when you have typed in the appropriate instruction the computer will display on the terminal screen the number of references available in your chosen area.

If you have chosen to investigate stab wounds of the chest and have typed in 'wound', you might be told there are 200–300

(continued)

references, or even more. This is an impossible amount of information to sort through, so you narrow or refine your field of search by entering 'stab'. (This is one area where the computer links themes.) This could still generate a large number of references, perhaps 80 or so. By being more specific still, refining the selection to 'chest', you might now be told that there are 20 references written in the last 5 years on stab wounds of the chest. This is a reasonable number of references to consider. By following the appropriate instructions you will be able to read the **abstract** (or summary) of each report. From this you can make a note of references that will be useful to you. Some libraries have the facility to print out the references you have chosen so that you have an accurate (and permanent) record from which to seek the article or book (Fig. 3.2).

You can see how time spent refining your ideas by discussion and identifying key words and synonyms pays dividends when you reach the computer. In some libraries the demand for computer searches is so great that time has to be booked and the length of time is limited. Thus it is essential to have carried out your preparatory clarification of ideas in order to utilise your available computer time to the full.

Many different organisations produce CD-ROMs. Some that you are most likely to come across in libraries are indicated below. However, with the rapid changes in information technology, there may be others in the future:

- **MEDLINE,** produced by the US National Library of Medicine, covers more than 4000 journals (including major nursing journals), and outlines over 11 million citations dating back to 1966.

- **CINAHL** (Cumulative Index to Nursing and Allied Health Literature) is also produced in the US, indexes over 500 journals and has more than 450 000 citations dating back to 1982. Approximately 30 000 records are added annually.

- RCN Nurse ROM was produced by the Royal College of Nursing. The fifth and final issue was released in March 1997.

```
Bookshelf                                    Catalogue Enquiry
                                             ===============
Print requested from port OPAC14; of search 'S* 9 & 19'
=================================================================
N. Author(s)  . . .Title...........................Class .......Location-status ..
1 BRADEN, B J    Predictive validity of
  BERGSTROM, N   the Braden Scale for
                 pressure sore risk in
                 a nursing home population.
                 (Research) Research in
                 Nursing and Health 17(6)
                 Dec 1994 459-470
2 BURD, C and    Skin care strategies in a
  others         skilled nursing home.
                 (Research on pressure
                 sore prevention and
                 treatment) Journal of
                 Gerontological Nursing
                 20(11) Nov 1994 28-34
3 ST CLAIR, M    Tissue Viability Society.
  and others     Measuring pressure sore
                 incidence: a study.
                 (Research) Nursing
                 Standard 9, 1 Feb 1995
                 50-51
4 SHIELDS, N     Journal of Wound Care
                 Nursing. Sore concerns.
                 (Survey of pressure sores
                 in nursing homes in the
                 Eastern HSS area in
                 Northern Ireland.
                 Research) Nursing Times
                 91, 1 Feb 1995 68, 70, 72
5 HALFENS, R J G Knowledge, beliefs and
                 use of nursing methods in
  EGGINK, M      preventing pressure sores
                 in Dutch hospitals.
                 (Research) International
                 Journal of Nursing
                 Studies 32(1) Feb 1995
                 16-26
6 BONNEFOY, M    Implication of cytokines
  and others     in the aggravation of
                 malnutrition and
                 hypercatabolism in
                 elderly patients with
                 severe pressure sores.
                 (Research) Age and Ageing
                 24(1) Jan 1995 37-42
```

Figure 3.2   Example of a printout from a literature search on pressure ulcers.

- **British Nursing Index** (BNI) started in January 1997 and consolidates *Nursing Bibliography*, RCN Nurse ROM and NMI (Nursing and Midwifery Index). The database includes over 220 health-related journals, many from the UK, and contains over 52 300 records. Approximately 9000 references are added each year. The BNI is produced in three formats: on the internet, by subscription (CD-ROM available quarterly), and in printed form, with 12 issues a year and an annual compendium.

- The **Cochrane Library** is a database updated by a team of over 7000 Cochrane Collaboration members from all over the world, organised into specialised review groups. Among the many components of this electronic publication are the Cochrane Database of Systematic Reviews, Abstracts of Reviews of Effectiveness and the Cochrane Controlled Trials Register.

Those with access to the **Internet** will find many **websites** very useful, such as the English National Board (ENB) home page. The ENB home page contains circulars, research papers, information leaflets and many other aspects relevant to nursing. If possible, check out too such home pages (and their associated links) as the Department of Health (DoH), United Kingdom Central Council (UKCC) and the National Institute for Clinical Excellence (NICE). Other examples include the RCN home page, home pages for journals and universities, and even departments within universities. Additionally, the internet can provide access to research and discussions of research, often from all over the world, especially the US.

If you lack the necessary abilities to undertake such a search, or are daunted or overwhelmed by the prospect, there is much useful guidance to be found. For example, see Ward's (2001) article on Internet skills for nurses, which provides a valuable hands-on introduction and overview; his home page is also a useful resource.

Comparisons have been made between the various databases available. Research has been carried out into the usefulness of MEDLINE and CINAHL in nursing literature searches. Brazier & Begley (1996) concluded that there was no difference in the two databases overall but that the references in MEDLINE were significantly more accessible in all aspects of nursing, except the organisation of nursing. Depending on your particular area of interest and geographical location, when comparing the BNI with CINAHL, you may find the BNI a more useful starting point. CINAHL is international and therefore has more scope. However, you might find it is less obtainable and has less relevance to nurses practising in the UK.

Further help

Currently, at least, it is important to note that not all journals are as yet indexed on the databases. (Check with the librarian, who might have a list of those that are excluded/included.) If you need to search the literature for information prior to the 1980s, a manual search will almost certainly be necessary using various indexes or specialised **abstracting journals**. Hence manual searching skills are still required. Again, the key words are helpful when you search abstracting journals. An abstracting journal is a publication that summarises published material in a particular subject area. For example, *Nursing Research Abstracts* was published by the Department of Health and Social Security four times a year. Many libraries will still have copies, although the last issue was volume 16, number 4 in 1994. Publication ceased because it was felt that CD-ROMs had made the abstracts obsolete. Prior to the release of the RCN Nurse CD-ROM, the information was contained in the *Nursing Bibliography*, which was published by the Royal College of Nursing every 2 months and listed published nursing texts. Not all the titles listed were research publications, so be careful if you are seeking research findings. Remember, too, that if the abstract is of potential interest you will need to seek out the original unabridged text to be able to evaluate the work in detail.

The library might offer a literature searching service for you (sometimes as part of your membership contract, sometimes at a nominal charge). If you are a member of the RCN the College Library will carry out a search for you if you cannot get to the library in person, although there might be a time delay depending on demand. If you are a student at university there are likely to be facilities available to you on the campus. However, Moorbath (1995) reports a worrying decline in access and availability of libraries to nurses. He concludes his study by saying that the number of specialised library sites has fallen over the last few years and in 20% of cases surveyed the distance between college sites and libraries is over 10 miles. However, in the remaining 80% there has been an improvement in facilities with access to new technologies. Moorbath states that the fewer remaining libraries have the opportunity to offer more professional services than small, unstaffed or partly staffed libraries. If you have to travel, make sure you are well organised and clear about what you wish to find out. Finally, ensure that your briefing is as precise as possible. Make it clear how far back you wish the search to go: just the last 5 years or the last 40? Make sure you stipulate which languages you are fluent in: failing to do this can be frustrating if your search generates articles in other than your native tongue(s).

Starting to read

Once you have four or five references, I suggest you start reading. Always read the most recent article or book first as there will be useful references taking you back through the literature to yet more references. Once your reading is underway you will soon find that the real problem is not difficulty in getting references but the potential for being overwhelmed by a pile of paper, and indeed being sidetracked. Again, your key words will help you keep to your original aim and you need to remember that time is a finite resource and needs managing. The next chapter considers how you can stay up to date with all the reading and information and make records of your findings. All the new references in this third edition have been taken from journals and material that were available in my local library. I have selected examples that are in nursing journals commonly held in libraries, so that you should be able to access them easily, although they do not necessarily represent the most in-depth or detailed study on the topic.

4

Making records

Key words:
■ References   ■ Bibliographic software

Whether you are reading in the comfort of your own home or in a library, it is wise to record details of what you are reading. However time-consuming or irritating this might seem, take care to record them accurately and comprehensively. This might seem a chore now but in a few weeks or months, when you come to write an essay, collate your references or share your information with others, you will be glad you spent the time!

Where to record these details

Your records can be handwritten or stored electronically. First, I will discuss using index cards and then look at how a hand-held or laptop computer can make life easier.

The written version

Lined index cards 20×12 cm (various sizes are available from most stationers) are a simple and efficient tool to record the necessary details. These should be stored somewhere safe and in alphabetical order by author(s) for easy retrieval. An old shoe box might be suitable storage or you can buy file boxes or drawers for your cards if you prefer. Index cards are small enough to carry around but large enough to contain essential information. Record each article or report on a separate card. Even record articles and reports you have looked at and decided are not relevant to your work now – they might be later! Or they might be useful to someone else.

Write your key words on one of the cards so that you have a written record of them to remind you of your original objective(s).

Information technology

Generating, storing and using recorded information is made easier if you have a hand-held (notebook or palmtop) or even laptop computer because you can enter data directly while reading. This can then be transferred to your home computer, where you can build up a bank of **references** and information that is quickly accessible and easily manipulated into various formats for essay and project writing. Commercial software packages such as Procite, Reference Manager and Endnote are available and compatible with various types of computers. This **bibliographic software** for personal collections of references has made the task of filing and searching for relevant references very easy. Most systems enable you to identify the references you require from those you have recorded and will format them in the style required by your college or publisher. (These differ, so to save time and anguish at a later date, always check out in advance what the 'house' format demands.) Some too (for example Endnote) will search online databases and organise their references, creating instant bibliographies. I have cited just three software packages that are available; however, information technology is a volatile market, which means rapid changes in **software** and **hardware** (the computer itself). Finally, an important point: remember to make a back-up copy on a floppy disk in case of computer failure or power cuts, which can cause havoc with some systems.

What information should be recorded

1 Author's surname and initials. These will be found on the title page (Fig. 4.1 (A)). If a book has chapters by different authors, the author's name will be given after the chapter title.

2 Editor's name and initials (if it is a book of chapters from different contributors) will be found on the title page (in this case the author and editor are the same person (Fig. 4.1 (B)).

3 Year published. This occurs on the bibliographic page, which is usually the reverse of the title page (Fig. 4.2 (C)). Note that it is the date of publication, *not* the date of the last reprint (i.e. in Fig. 4.2, (C) not (D)).

4 Title of book and subtitles (Fig. 4.1 (E)).

5 Edition, if not the first (Fig. 4.1 (F)).

(E) # OGIER'S READING RESEARCH

How to make research
more approachable

(F) **THIRD EDITION**

(B) Edited by

(A) ## Nicky Lanoë

RGN, RCNT, RNT, MSc, ILTM
Freelance Lecturer/Consultant
St Martins, Guernsey, Channel Islands

Foreword by

Margaret E Ogier

RGN, RM, DipN, RNT, BSc, PhD, C Psychol
Freelance Lecturer/Researcher
Castel, Guernsey, Channel Islands

(G) 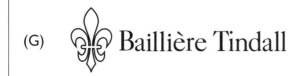 Baillière Tindall

Figure 4.1   Sample title page.

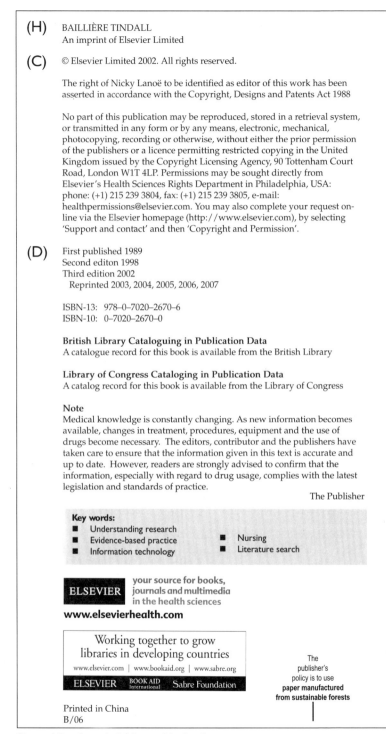

(H)   BAILLIÈRE TINDALL
An imprint of Elsevier Limited

(D)   First published 1989
Second editon 1998
Third edition 2002
   Reprinted 2003, 2004, 2005, 2006, 2007

ISBN-13:   978–0–7020–2670–6
ISBN-10:   0–7020–2670–0

British Library Cataloguing in Publication Data
A catalogue record for this book is available from the British Library

Library of Congress Cataloging in Publication Data
A catalog record for this book is available from the Library of Congress

Note
Medical knowledge is constantly changing. As new information becomes available, changes in treatment, procedures, equipment and the use of drugs become necessary. The editors, contributor and the publishers have taken care to ensure that the information given in this text is accurate and up to date. However, readers are strongly advised to confirm that the information, especially with regard to drug usage, complies with the latest legislation and standards of practice.

The Publisher

Key words:
- Understanding research
- Evidence-based practice
- Information technology
- Nursing
- Literature search

ELSEVIER   your source for books, journals and multimedia in the health sciences
www.elsevierhealth.com

Working together to grow libraries in developing countries
www.elsevier.com | www.bookaid.org | www.sabre.org
ELSEVIER   BOOK AID International   Sabre Foundation

The publisher's policy is to use paper manufactured from sustainable forests

Printed in China
B/06

Figure 4.2   Sample bibliographic detail page.

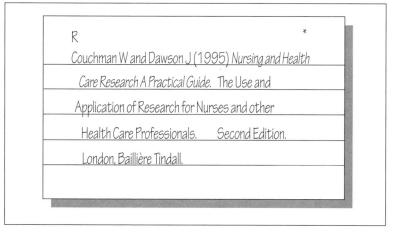

R   *

Couchman W and Dawson J (1995) Nursing and Health

Care Research A Practical Guide. The Use and

Application of Research for Nurses and other

Health Care Professionals.   Second Edition.

London, Baillière Tindall.

Figure 4.3   Completed record card for a book reference.

6 Number of pages, if only part of a book is used.

7 Place of publication and publisher (Figs 4.1 (G) and 4.2 (H)).

Figure 4.3 shows an example of a completed record card.

The procedure is a little more detailed for articles in journals:

1 Author's surname and initials.

2 Year of publication.

3 Title of article and subtitles.

4 Journal title.

5 Volume and part numbers.

6 The inclusive page numbers of the article.

7 Date of publication.

Figure 4.4 shows an example of a completed record card for a journal article; and look at the Reference and Further Reading sections towards the end of this book for further examples.

A tip that you might find useful, whether you are using manual or computer recording, is to note where you obtained the reference, journal article or book. I use the right-hand corner of the index card for this (see Figs 4.3 and 4.4). If it is my own copy I use an asterisk, if I borrowed it from a friend or colleague I put their name; if I obtained it from a library, I put the

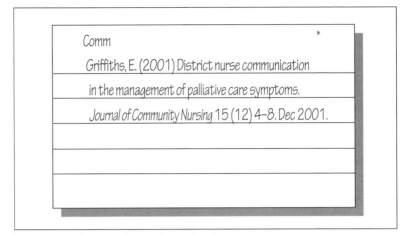

Figure 4.4   Completed record card for a journal reference.

library's name. If it is a library copy, besides putting the name or initials of the library you borrowed it from (e.g. Royal College of Nursing, RCN), you can also put the class and accession numbers. This might seem like a lot of extra work before you .even start the task of reading, but in 2 or 3 months' time when you refer to your cards and want more details on a particular aspect you can retrieve the original report without too much difficulty.

The final piece of information to be recorded on the card must wait until you have read the article or report. You can then use the top left-hand corner to indicate the subject matter of the article, e.g. 'man' to indicate 'management', 'n man' to indicate 'nursing management', etc. You can use any categories that are relevant to you. Use one of your cards to record your abbreviations, otherwise when you return to your cards after a few months you might not remember whether 'cc' stands for 'catheter care' or 'coronary care'. Similar information can be stored on computer, depending on what software you are using.

All this takes time but, in the long term, it will allow you to retrieve articles if you want to refresh your memory on some aspect or find information for an essay or project. In this respect, information technology will help you greatly.

As noted earlier, your course director or publisher will usually stipulate the way you are required to reference your work.

There are two frequently used referencing systems. The first is called the Harvard system, which is used in this book: the author's name and date appear in the text, with the full references in alphabetical order (under the author's family name) at the end of the chapter or book. The other is called the Vancouver system: a number is placed in the text where a reference occurs, with the references listed in numerical order at the end of the chapter or book. Be cautious, though; adaptations exist of both of these formats. For example, in some modified versions of the Harvard system, page numbers for direct quotes are also required in the text.

With all this work completed you can now start to read and appraise your chosen report. Chapters 5–9 consider sections of the report, as you are likely to encounter them.

5
Making sense of reports

Key words:
- Abstract   - Report layout

Before you can get to grips with a more in-depth analysis of the constituents of the research process that are discussed in the next few chapters, you first need to be able to make sense of what you are reading. Depending on the subject matter and the purpose of the activity, you are likely to employ different reading strategies. For example, if I am reading a fictional novel or tabloid newspaper I tend to focus on aspects that are of particular interest and skim read the rest. I also adopt a different attitude to what I am reading. In the examples used, I certainly would not expect to believe everything that is in print! To a certain extent, scepticism is a healthy trait to develop, whatever and however you are approaching the task. Certainly, consumption of inaccurate or unsound research findings can be hazardous to health.

It is far easier to read something if you have some general idea of what it is about, an overview of the whole. Authors of research reports are aware of this and want to attract the reader, so they usually preface the report with an **abstract** (a summary of why the study was done and the main results). If you are reading a journal article, the abstract usually takes the form of a paragraph at the start of the article. Such paragraphs are often set in a different typeface to attract your attention (Fig. 5.1). In theses and research reports, the first page is usually devoted to the abstract.

Read the abstract through several times to get an idea of what you are about to read. If you are using your own copy, you might like to underline or highlight key words. If you are

PERGAMON

International Journal of Nursing Studies 39 (2002) 17–26

INTERNATIONAL JOURNAL OF
NURSING
STUDIES

www.elsevier.com/locate/ijnurstu

A qualitative study of the theoretical models used by UK mental health nurses to guide their assessments with family caregivers of people with dementia

Angela Carradice[a],*, Marie Claire Shankland[b,1], Nigel Beail[c]

[a] University of Sheffield, UK
[b] Community Health Sheffield, National Health Service Trust, UK
[c] University of Sheffield, Western Bank, Sheffield, South Yorkshire, S10 2TP, UK

Received 7 July 2000; received in revised form 20 November 2000; accepted 11 January 2001

Abstract

Some researchers suggest that nurse training does not provide adequate theoretical knowledge to guide mental health nurses' work with carers of people with dementia. In recent years theoretical guidance for working with carers has emerged in the nursing literature. However, little attention has been given to theory practice links. This study used interpretative phenomenological analysis to investigate the theoretical model used by nurses to guide carer assessments. During the analysis the data evolved into a description of the model underlying the nurses' work. In the discussion this model was compared with the stress process model (SPM). This comparison highlighted striking similarities between the themes in the nurses' model of carer stress and the theoretical constructs of the SPM. However, the SPM describes influential links between different constructs which were absent in the nurses' model. The research illustrates developmental training needs for mental health nursing to improve the efficacy of assessments and therefore, interventions. © 2001 Elsevier Science Ltd. All rights reserved.

Keywords: Mental health nurses; Assessment and theoretical model

1. Introduction

Due to social and political changes in the UK more family caregivers for people with dementia are being referred to mental health nurses for assessment and treatment. Caregiving for a member of the family who is

suffering from dementia can be stressful (Schulz et al., 1990). Accepting the view that theory should guide practice (Holdsworth, 1995), it is recommended that assessments of carers should be based on a theoretical understanding of the stress process of caring. However, nurse training does not provide the required theoretical knowledge to guide the nurses' work (Sheppard, 1991). Sheppard (1991) explained that the gap between what nurses know and the demands of their role exists because nursing theory is inadequate. This means that nurses' work is developed by trial and error experience, rather than theoretical training. One concern is that if the theoretical models adopted by the nurses are limited and fragmentary as suggested by Sheppard (1991), then the practice may mirror this. Without comprehensive assessment based on some

*Corresponding author. Forest Lodge, 5 Forest Close, Sheffield S35 0JW, UK. Tel.: +44-114-2716078; fax: +44-114-2716086.

E-mail address: angelac@chsheff-tr.trent.nhs.uk (A. Carradice).

[1] Also at Clinical Psychology Department, Northern General Hospital, Herries Road, Sheffield, South Yorkshire, S5 7AU, UK.

Figure 5.1   Abstract (from Carradice A, Shankland MC, Beail N 2001 A qualitative study of the theoretical models used by UK mental health nurses to guide their assessments with family caregivers of people with dementia. International Journal of Nursing Studies 39(1): 17–26. Reproduced with permission of Elsevier Science Ltd).

using a borrowed copy, write the key words on your index card or enter them into your computerised record.

If you are still not sure what the report is about, check any difficult terms or phrases. It can also be useful to turn to the end of the article and read the conclusion or summary several times, again identifying key words. Remember that researchers have a responsibility to write in an engaging manner, clearly describing and expressing their approach and findings in order to appeal to practitioners and other allied professionals. If this is not achieved it might in itself be an indication of the overall 'quality' of the report, if not the research itself.

Now, hopefully, you have some idea about the report, but do *not* be tempted to think that this is enough and you can skip the tedious bit in the middle! If you do, you might find that you have come to the wrong conclusions. For the next part, bring your knowledge and common sense into play and use the pointers provided in this book to help you read critically and with purpose. You need to use your own experience and knowledge to formulate questions about what you are reading.

Pathways and stepping stones through a research report

There is generally a common structure or format to research reports, although this can vary slightly, sometimes because of the research approach (**qualitative** or **quantitative research**) employed and sometimes because of the 'house' rules of the publication. Either way, the most common elements to explore are as follows.

see
Chapter 7

The first two parts (which we have already mentioned) are the *title*, followed by the *abstract*. The other sections or parts of a report are listed here to give you an overall picture; each part is the subject of a separate chapter in its own right:

- *Introduction.* This gives the background to the study and tells you why the particular piece of research was undertaken. A brief résumé of previous and related work will also be given, either in the introduction or possibly under a separate heading, **Literature Review**, which will be helpful to you with your own literature search as the background literature is discussed.

see
Chapter 6

see
Chapter 7
■ *Method or Methodology*. This is an account of how the study was carried out.

see
Chapter 8
■ *Results*. This is usually a short factual section in which the findings of the study are depicted. Quantitative studies often use graphs and tables to clarify and expand on the statistical findings. Qualitative results are less likely to benefit from such treatment because, although no less rigorous, they tend to focus on the rich descriptive material that has been collected, often using direct quotations from **participants**.

see
Chapter 9
■ *Discussion*. In this section the author discusses the findings of the study in the light of previous work described in the introduction/literature review, and other relevant issues.

see
Chapter 9
■ *Conclusion*. The author summarises the study, drawing the threads together and perhaps indicating the strengths, weaknesses and implications for use of the study.

■ *References*. All studies mentioned in the text should be listed in detail. You should be able to access any of these relatively easily if the references have been presented correctly.

■ *Appendices* contain material of interest relevant to the study itself but not included in the body of the report (e.g. the questionnaire or interview schedule used during the research).

You now have an overview of the **layout** or order of presentation of a research report. Depending on whether you are reading an article in a journal or an original thesis, you will find that the parts vary in the amount of detail covered (ranging from a few lines to several chapters) but the basic format will be the same. However, you should be aware of the enormous difference in depth and detail between a thesis and a 2000-word report written for publication in a journal. If the article is based on a thesis, the full document will be cited in the references or acknowledged in a note at the beginning of the article.

The headings in a report are an important guide to answering the essential question: Is this an account of a research study or is it merely someone else's views and opinions? There are many interesting, well-informed journal articles and books written by well-known authors, but however good they might be they are not necessarily research reports. If you have been asked to write a critique of a piece of research, or if you are using evidence to justify a nursing decision or action, you need to know if what you are reading is an actual research report or merely a knowledgeable account of facts and opinions that perhaps reflects currently available evidence. Any material that fits clearly into the headings in the bullet list above is likely to be a piece of research. This distinction is important as nursing moves forwards to become an evidence-based profession. You need to be able to make firm judgements about the quality of the research, the appropriateness of the techniques used and the veracity of the writer's conclusions. These are skills you need to develop and I hope that by the time you have read the research, with this book as a guide, you will be more informed and critical in your reading. This is not to imply that a key purpose of reading research is to fault-find or criticise as such. Rather, being critical in this context means reading consciously in an insightful, sensitive and professional manner.

To help clarify your thoughts, prepare an A4 summary sheet with the headings shown in Fig. 5.2. You might feel that this is duplicating your index card. However, when you start reading research reports you might have difficulty picking out the salient points so that they fit on to the index card. You can summarise the points on the A4 sheet and transpose them to the index card at the end of the exercise. Alternatively, you could log them on an electronically prepared template.

Developing a questioning attitude to what you read

Now that you have read the abstract and the conclusions, you should have an idea of what the study is about. Earlier I warned you to be careful not to fall into the trap of thinking that this will be enough.

Completing the first part of the summary sheet with the title, author and date of publication should be easy enough. What might not be immediately apparent, however, is the date when the study was actually carried out (as opposed to the publication date of the report). The date of the study might only become apparent as you read the introduction. On occasions, the only way I have discovered when the work was done was from material in the appendices, such as dated letters or

RESEARCH REPORT SUMMARY

Title of study:

Authors:

Date of study: Date of publication:

Aim of study:

Research questions and/or hypotheses:

Sample and sample size:

Method of study and research tools used:

Results:

Conclusions of the study:

Figure 5.2   Research report summary form.

questionnaires. You might wonder why it is important to be concerned about when exactly the research was done. This is because there is always a gap between writing and publishing, often as long as 18 months to 2 years, and there might have been an even longer gap between completion of the research and the writing of the report or article! Some areas of nursing

RESEARCH REPORT SUMMARY

Title of study: A qualitative study of the theoretical models used by UK mental health nurses to guide their assessments with family caregivers of people with dementia.

Authors: Carradice A., Shankland M.C. and Beail N.

Date of study: 7th July 2000. **Date of publication:** 2001

Aim of study: To investigate the theoretical model used by nurses to guide carer assessments.

Research questions and/or hypotheses: Not given, inferred in the aim.

Sample and sample size: Not apparent from abstract.

Method of study and research tools used: Interpretative phenomenology, the evolving data being used to describe the model underlying the mental health nurses' work.

Discussion: The model in practice was compared to the previously identified stress process model (SPM). Major similarities were found between the SPM and current practice, though some links between different constructs were absent.

Conclusions: Highlights developmental needs for nurses to improve their assessment skills and thus interventions.

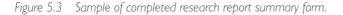

Figure 5.3   Sample of completed research report summary form.

are changing quickly, such as the facilities for day surgery or non-invasive investigations, so the information in the report could be out of date before it is published, or it might have been superseded by more up-to-date knowledge. This does *not* mean that the report should not be read – there is still a possibility that it will provide valuable insights. However, it *does* mean that if you are considering implementing the findings or changing your practice as a result of your reading, you must be aware of how current the research actually is.

An example of a completed summary sheet for the journal article used in Fig. 5.1 is shown in Fig. 5.3.

Each of the following chapters (6–9) addresses a section of the research report. As you should always be prepared to ask questions about what you are reading, some questions are given in each chapter to help get you started.

Special terms, used in research reports in a more precise manner than in general speech, are set in bold type and are defined in the Glossary. Not all the terms will be found in any one report and not all possible terms are covered in this book. However, more detailed texts are suggested in the Further Reading at the end of this book.

6

The introduction and literature review

Key words:
- Literature review
- Hypothesis
- Null hypothesis

The introduction usually includes a statement of why the research was done. The **literature review** gives an overview of previous research or writings on the topic. In a research report or thesis this will form a separate chapter/section but in a journal article it is covered in the first few paragraphs.

As mentioned in Chapter 5, there are essential questions a reader needs to ask to develop skills of critical appraisal, for example: see Chapter 5

- What was the aim of the study?

Fill this in on your A4 summary sheet (see Figs 5.2 and 5.3). You will need to refer to the aim several times while you are reading to remind yourself what the researcher was trying to study. For instance, when you get to the results section, do the results agree with the aim? And you will need to check the aim against the conclusions. You might even want to refer to the aim while reading the methodology and consider whether you would have used the same processes to find answers to the stipulated purpose of the study.

Spend a few minutes at this point thinking about what other questions you need to be asking yourself about the introduction and aim(s) of the study. Make full use of your experience, knowledge and common sense, as outlined in Chapter 5. Don't be afraid to be naïve; questioning what might seem like the obvious helps to remove professional 'blinkers'. For example, does the introduction outline the context of the study, clarify the

see Chapter 5

research problem to be explored and provide a rationale for this, and clarify key terms? Overall, therefore (in your opinion), was there value in undertaking the study at all?

The literature review usually presents studies and reports that have informed the researcher and provides the background or foundation upon which the present study is based. The literature review leads into either the research questions (an early indicator that the research **method** is going to veer towards a qualitative approach) or hypotheses (more indicative of a quantitative approach). Ask yourself whether you consider the review to be comprehensive – are you aware of other work in the field that should have been considered? The nature of the sources too can be of importance. Primary sources are those that the author has accessed and read directly, secondary sources are cited from these. Logically, more credibility is attached to the former, as inaccuracies can occur when reproducing material. It is also important to note how the literature was explored – merely described and summarised, or critically reviewed.

Another useful question to ask yourself is:

■ What was the research question being asked?

see
Chapter 1 At the beginning of this book, we examined the aim of Ogier's (1982) research study, which was about the influence of ward sisters on student nurses. After discussion, the research question was developed into a form for which answers could be sought. The research was a descriptive study to find out about ward sister–student nurse interactions. As the study progressed and answers began to form in response to the research questions, so it became possible to formulate hypotheses.

Hypothesis

A **hypothesis** (plural, hypotheses) is a statement that is based on knowledge or information and which has yet to be proved or disproved, supported or rejected. In a seminal piece of nursing research, Boore (1978) gives two experimental hypotheses:

1 'The preoperative giving of information about postoperative treatment and care, and teaching exercises to be performed postoperatively, will minimise the rise in biochemical indicators of stress.'

2 'A relationship will be demonstrated between the measurements of biochemical indicators of stress and some other indicators of patient welfare.'

Null hypothesis

A **null hypothesis** states that there will be *no significant difference* between the control and the experimental groups. Using an experimental research design, the researcher sets out to gather data that will support or reject this hypothesis. For example, Kerr et al (1996) used an experimental design to study whether providing parents with advice in the postnatal period would reduce sleep problems in infants. Their null hypothesis was that 'there was no statistically significant difference in the sleeping behaviour of the control group and the intervention group'. The null hypothesis was rejected. Therefore, advice in the postnatal period *does* appear to be beneficial in preventing sleep problems in infants.

Be careful when you are reading your research report, as it is easy to come to the wrong conclusion. If the experimental hypothesis is supported, the meaning will be exactly opposite to what it would be if the null hypothesis was supported. In both the Boore (1978) and Kerr et al (1996) studies the hypotheses were supported, which means that preoperative information *does* minimise the biochemical indicators of stress and that postnatal advice *does* reduce sleep problems in infants. A study by Sleep (1988), investigating whether salt in the bath affected the healing of episiotomies, found that 90% of mothers found no difference whether they used salt or not. In Sleep's study the null hypothesis was supported, showing that salt in bath water does *not* significantly affect wound healing. So be careful with your reading and check which hypothesis has been supported.

Further questions to ask yourself are:

- In the study you are reading, has the researcher posed a hypothesis?
- Is the hypothesis relevant to the question being asked or to the aim of the study?

Not all research studies have hypotheses. This is influenced predominately by the research **method** that is adopted, which in turn should be influenced by the aim, i.e. what it is that the research sets out to explore. Ogier's (1982) study employed a grounded theory approach. As the name suggests, this approach is grounded in the real world, seeking to observe life experiences. The researcher sets out to collect and analyse qualitative data with the aim of developing theories and propositions. Hence it is categorised as inductive reasoning, as it works from specific observations to more general thinking about an issue. (Conversely, quantitative studies adopt deductive reasoning – working from general observations and breaking them down into their constituent parts.) Ogier's (1982) work therefore started with the aim of describing what sisters were doing to improve or impede learning in the clinical area. Only as the study advanced and differences between medical and surgical ward sisters became apparent did Ogier formulate a hypothesis. Grahn & Danielson (1996), evaluating an education and support programme for cancer patients, also used a grounded theory approach to their descriptive study because they felt it was a research design sensitive to the topic and where testing hypotheses would be inappropriate. Chapter 7 considers different ways of carrying out research in order to meet the aims of the study, in other words the method or methodology.

7

The method or methodology

Key words:

- Ethics
- Quantitative research
- Qualitative research
- Descriptive research
  - *Cross-sectional study*
  - *Longitudinal study*
- Experimental research
  - *Groups*
    - Experimental
    - Control
  - *Variables*
    - Independent
    - Dependent

- *Randomised controlled trial*
- Action research
- Sample
- Research tools
  - *Reliability*
  - *Validity*
- Interviews
  - *Structured*
  - *Semi-structured*
  - *Open ended*

Both **method** and **methodology** relate to the way in which the researcher tried to fulfil the aim of the study you have just identified in the report you are reading. In Chapter 2 the philosophy underpinning the 'new' NHS was discussed. This reasoned way of thinking must also be evident in the methodology chosen by the researcher: was the method employed appropriate to the purpose of the research? Methodology includes such aspects as **research design** used, **sample** size and selection, **research tools** used and ways of collecting and analysing data. You might also at this point think about the **ethics** and ethical considerations and implications of the research you are studying (see, for example, de Raeve 1996).

see Chapter 2

There are various ways of classifying research but perhaps the most helpful approach is to consider the three main types of research that you are likely to encounter:

G ▶ ■ **descriptive research**

G ▶ ■ **experimental research**

G ▶ ■ **action research.**

Within these frameworks you will also encounter research that is quantitative or qualitative or a mixture of both. There is no shortage of articles and discussion on the pros and cons of each type of research, so follow these up as appropriate for further details.

Quantitative research is concerned with collecting and analysing data that focus on numbers and frequencies, seeking to establish cause and effect, rather than on meaning or experience. This type of research is mainly associated with experimental designs such as those used by Kerr et al (1996). Hsu & Gallinagh (2001) used such an approach to explore the relationships between health beliefs and utilisation of free health examinations in older people living in Taiwan. They sought to establish statistically significant differences between users and non-users.

Qualitative research is mainly descriptive and involves the collection and analysis of data concerned with meanings, attitudes and beliefs, rather than data that result in numerical counts from which statistical inferences can be drawn. The see
Chapter 6 example used in Chapter 6 regarding grounded theory relates to just such an approach. For other examples, see the studies by Waterman et al (1996), who evaluated the introduction of case management on a newly created rehabilitation floor at an elderly care hospital, or Spouse (1990), who sought ways of improving the quality of the learning environment for student nurses in clinical areas. In Sweden, Hansebo & Kihlgren (2001) explored carers' reflections about their interactions with patients suffering from severe dementia.

Qualitative research tends to generate a lot of evidence gathered through a variety of means. This too requires analysis, and this can be problematical: how do you analyse people's opinions, for example? Russell & Gregory (1993) have produced some answers to this question that include both manual and information technology methods, but such detailed discussion is beyond the scope of this book. However, although there are many different approaches to gathering and analysing qualitative data, the processes involved tend to follow a similar format. As with quantitative analysis, they reflect the need to proceed in a rigorous, logical and systematic manner, with the purpose of discovering underlying patterns and dimensions of relationships and behaviour. If you are reading a piece of qualitative research, determine which form or forms of analysis were used and explore the philosophy, method and process of this in more depth.

Some researchers use both quantitative and qualitative methods and it is not always easy to determine which, if either method, predominates. For example, the study by Barrett et al (1996) used a descriptive design that included both quantitative and qualitative data to evaluate a baccalaureate nursing programme. So did the semi-quantitative descriptive investigation undertaken by Mutasa (2001), which analysed risk factors associated with non-compliance with methadone substitution therapy in a community in outer London. Another study (Moon & Cho 2001) used physiological measurements of stress alongside self-rating scales and interviews to determine the effects of handholding on anxiety in patients undergoing cataract surgery under local anaesthesia.

One method is not better than another; what is important is that the method of research most appropriate to the aim of the study is chosen, and that – subsequently – a logical, deduced method of data analysis is applied. This is where your knowledge and nursing experience are invaluable as you question whether the method chosen seems to be the sensible choice. Russell & Gregory (1993) comment that qualitative research has 'come of age' and that it is now accepted that qualitative research can be an end in itself not just the prelude to a 'proper' quantitative study.

- Is the report you are reading quantitative, qualitative or a mixture of both approaches? Remember, as stated before, this is not always as obvious as it may first appear.

Descriptive research

Within this framework the researcher tries to describe accurately (to paint a picture in words and figures) the findings derived from careful, systematic collection and recording of information or data. Many nursing studies are descriptive. Nursing research is still 'young' and there are many aspects of nursing that need to be studied and described. The different ways data are gathered are numerous and often referred to as research tools; these include **questionnaires**, **interviews** and **observations**. The different types of tool, together with their advantages and disadvantages, are discussed in more detail later in the chapter. First, some different descriptive studies are explained briefly to show how these techniques can be used to inform nurses.

Atkinson & Sklaroff (1987) studied the care provided for 75 physically disabled patients admitted to acute general hospital wards. They were also interested to see how hospitalisation had affected their well-being on return home. The study shows that the layout of the wards, nursing routines and inadequate nurse–patient communication resulted in the disabled patients being more dependent than they need have been.

Barrett et al (1996) wanted to find out if graduates from a nursing programme felt they had achieved their end-of-course objectives and whether those objectives met the employer's needs. By analysing the responses of the students and employers they were able to conclude the course was satisfactory.

Coates (1985) used a descriptive **cross-sectional** study to examine the nutritional status of patients in wards that were organised differently (rather than patients in the same ward over months or years). Hicks et al (1996) used semi-structured interviews to gather information about attitudes to research from six members of four primary health teams, again obtaining a cross-section of opinions.

Rather than using a cross-sectional design, some researchers use **longitudinal** studies that examine the same group of people over time. Kirkevold et al (1996) used a short time-span (8 weeks) when they studied the recovery of heart surgery patients, whereas Jerrett & Costello (1996) spent 2 years gathering data from parents of asthmatic children and describing how they did or did not gain control of the situation.

Experimental research

This type of research is useful for establishing a relationship between cause and effect. In Chapter 6, we looked at two studies that used experimental design when considering hypotheses: both Boore (1978) and Kerr et al (1996) used an experimental design to see whether information-giving would result in a reduced problem, i.e. postoperative stress and sleep problems in infants, respectively.

see
Chapter 6

It is usual when embarking on an experimental research project to divide the group of people or things – the **participants** or **sample** – into subgroups that are as similar as possible. One subgroup, the **experimental group**, experiences the factor under consideration. The second subgroup, the **control group**, does *not* experience the particular factor. If the two groups do not differ in any other way, any change that occurs in the experimental group but *not* in the control group would appear to be due to the introduced factor. This factor is referred to as a **variable**.

The **independent variable** is the experimental factor that is deliberately manipulated. In Boore (1978) and Kerr et al (1996), the independent variable was the level of information given to the experimental group but not to the control group.

The **dependent variable** is the aspect being studied to see if the experimental factor has any effect. In Boore (1978) the dependent variable was postoperative stress while in Kerr et al (1996) it was the sleep problems of infants.

When you are reading reports of experimental research it is important to remember what the variables are. One way of doing this is to write each one out on a card, labelling them independent or dependent, and then to use the card as a benchmark as you read through the report. When presenting results or discussing their findings, many authors refer to dependent or independent variables (but not what they were), so you frequently have to refer back to make sure you are not getting confused. Writing the variables on a card saves time and reduces your frustration levels! The study of Kerr et al (1996) is examined briefly below.

An example of an experimental study is Kerr et al (1996). One of the most common problems that causes parents of young

(continued)

children to seek advice from health professionals is the sleepless preschool child. Disturbed sleep puts the parents under stress and, in some cases, places the child at risk of abuse.

Kerr et al wanted to find out if health education could reduce the incidence of sleep problems. Participants were randomly allocated to either the control group (which contained 90 subjects) or the intervention – experimental – group (which contained 100 subjects); hence the term **randomised controlled trial**. The intervention group was given specific information on sleep patterns and settling methods when babies were 3 months old. The sleeping behaviour of both groups was compared 6 months later when the babies were 9 months old. Babies in the intervention group were sleeping better, with fewer problems, than babies in the control group.

- What are the variables being considered in Kerr et al's study? (See the end of this chapter, on page 59, for the answer.)

Action research

Action research and change are inextricably linked. In action research, the researcher pays attention to a particular problem, or perhaps a perceived change event, in a specific situation. It is a democratic and participatory approach in which the researcher works with staff (and sometimes co-researchers) to bring about change while at the same time fostering a climate of ownership and empowerment. The researcher observes in a systematic manner the way the problem is solved (or the change is implemented). A useful article by Waterman (1995) considers the differences between, and similarities of, 'traditional' and action research. The following examples of action research studies might help to clarify this research design or method.

Fretwell (1982) carried out a descriptive study in which she identified wards that were good teaching wards for student nurses and those that were less good. She followed this up with an action research study in which she developed a programme, based in the wards, to help sisters who had problems creating a learning environment in the clinical area. In this way she introduced change, watched and documented what happened, and reported it in *Freedom to change* (Fretwell 1985).

Since Fretwell's pioneering work with action research in nursing during the 1980s, other nurse researchers have used this method with success in a variety of nursing areas. West (1992) used an action research framework to change nursing staff's management of pressure ulcers into a research-based approach, which focused on the nutrition of the elderly. East & Robinson (1994) considered how best to bring about change, especially at ward level, and chose an action research design. The study identified that general managers and professionals have different agendas for change but there was common ground. Newton (1995) reviewed the use of action research in nursing and used action research to look at the effects of the care planning element of the computerised integrated Hospital Information System (HIS) on ward nurses in a district general hospital.

It can be seen from these examples that the use of action research is increasing and is particularly useful in areas related to change. Waterman (1995) provides a starting point for those interested in such a debate and draws on various schema (patterns) and criteria from which to judge the functionality and effectiveness of action research. The journal *Nurse Researcher*, volume 2, number 3, published March 1995, is devoted to a discussion of this topic and enables you to identify further references if you are particularly interested in this method of research.

Ethnography and phenomenology

As nursing attempts to move closer to becoming a research-based profession and to use evidence-based practice, so the types of design used in nursing research increase. For instance, you might come across reports such as Jan Savage's *Nursing intimacy: an ethnographic approach to nurse–patient interaction* (Savage 1995). This study explores what nurses understand by the notion of 'closeness' and assesses the support they might need where 'close' relationships with patients are encouraged. So how did Savage carry out the study and what does **ethnography** mean? There are various definitions; fortunately, Ballie (1995) has provided a comprehensive review of the origins and development of ethnography as a research approach in nursing. In essence, ethnography is a flexible method in which the researcher participates in people's lives, collecting data in order to provide an explanation for the chosen topic. Ethnography focuses on understanding the perspectives of the people being studied and observes them in everyday life rather than in artificial or experimental conditions.

> For example, I used an ethnographic approach (Lanoë 1994) when conducting the research for my Master of Science degree. I wanted to describe the extent to which primary nurses in a specific ward setting were aware of research in practice and establish any barriers or deficits that existed for them in terms of their knowledge, skills or attitudes. The focus was on describing their actual practice, the 'real' situation, their opinions, their experience, and so on.

Whereas the above is basically a descriptive methodology, **phenomenology** is an interpretative methodology that examines subjects' perceptions of their own experiences. The researcher attempts to present these perceptions with clarity and to interpret their structure and meaning. Phenomenology is a qualitative approach to research and, for some, is still controversial. However, as it records the subject's perceptions, it could be a valuable way of studying patients, their needs and nursing care.

> For example, the study by Hansebo & Kihlgren (2001) (see p. 42) used just such an approach to effect when considering the developmental needs of carers.

If you want to know more, Hallett (1995) is a most useful article. In the future there will be yet more research designs introduced for you to come to terms with, but for the moment we have looked at the main current designs that you will encounter in your reading.

- What type of research was carried out in the report you are reading? Remember to fill in your summary sheet.

Sample and sample size

After defining the research questions and choosing an appropriate type of research method, the author will need to decide on a **sample** and on the size of the sample. Again, both of these should be logically influenced by the research questions and the research design chosen. A sample is a selection of people from the possible **population**, e.g. 8 ward managers from a total of 24 managers working in hospital A.

The systematic selection of a sample to ensure that all possible members of the population stand an equal chance of being selected is known as a **random sampling**. For example, if all 24 ward managers were willing to take part in the study but time and money meant that only 8 could take part, then to ensure that each had a chance of being chosen all their names would be written on pieces of paper and put into a hat and 8 pieces of paper drawn out. Thus each manager would have an equal chance of being selected.

- What was the sample size in the report you are reading? Remember to fill in your summary sheet.

- What percentage is the sample size with relation to the possible population?

An example showing the importance of sample size is shown below.

> Six patients with anxiety neurosis were observed for half a day when there were forty similar patients attending the same day clinic.

- What was the significance of the length of time for which they were observed?

- Was it long enough?
- Was there any special significance to the date chosen?
- Was there a marked deviation from the usual routine that day?

If the aim of the study was to observe whether variation in routine caused an increase in a particular behaviour in specific patients, then the number and date chosen might be appropriate. However, if the aim of the study was to describe typical daily activities of patients with anxiety neurosis on a typical day, then the sample size and timing could be questioned.

So you can see why it is important for you to establish the aim of the study, as it has implications for the methods used, sample size, method of data collection, and so on. Some examples of the sample size used in different studies are shown below.

Ragneskog et al (1996) used video observation of five demented patients to assess the effect of music on their behaviour. Just five patients provided a lot of qualitative data. Using data that had been collected for an antenatal care project, Clement et al (1996) analysed 1882 maternity records, whereas Runciman et al (1996) looked at 414 patients over 75 years of age who attended an accident and emergency department and considered the effects of health visitor intervention.

So, in essence, a sample is a selection from the possible population of participants – the sampling frame. This selection, however, can be problematic in itself because it potentially can introduce sampling bias if the population chosen is not representative of the population from which it is drawn. Random sampling tends to be the most appropriate technique to employ for quantitative approaches seeking to establish cause and effect. Qualitative methodologies, however, predominantly need to take a more purposeful approach. They need to select a sample that includes credible and knowledgeable participants in the area of study.

Volume 3, number 4 of *Nurse Researcher* (June 1996) is devoted to sampling. If you feel in doubt about the size or selection of the sample in the report you are reading then you can find more detailed accounts of many aspects of sampling in this special issue, although some of the articles are rather complex.

Figure 7.1 depicts the methodological issues related to quantitative and qualitative research.

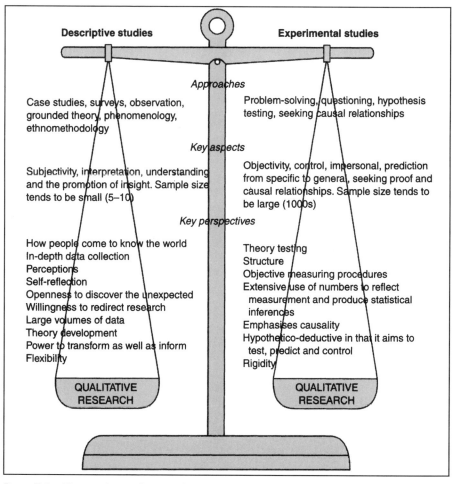

Figure 7.1   The weighting of various factors towards qualitative or quantitative research. This is depicted as a set of pan scales because there is no rigid divide between the two approaches, but rather a changing balance between the varying philosophies of research and the methods employed.

Pilot study

A preliminary study, or **pilot study**, will usually be carried out to test the proposed method and research tools for the main study. Sometimes this pilot study will be described in the methodology section, or it can provide enough material for a journal article in its own right, e.g. Dubyna & Quinn (1996) and Stonehouse & Butcher (1996).

The pilot study might identify problems in the choice of method or in the research tools, necessitating a change of plans. The purpose of the pilot study, therefore, is to refine the method and tools prior to the main study. You are likely to come across explanations of these pilot studies in full research reports, which should inform you of any alterations made, but not necessarily in journal articles. This is another good reason to make sure you read the whole report, not just the summary and the conclusions!

Research tools

These include questionnaires, audio and video recordings, interview schedules or observations. Observations can be behavioural or physiological (such as weight or skinfold thickness), participant or non-participant.

Participant observation is when the researcher is also part of what is being observed, a member of the team, e.g. when a staff nurse practising in a surgical ward observes the number of times student nurses spontaneously initiate conversation with patients aged over 70 years.

Non-participant observation is when the researcher is not directly part of the situation being observed – in essence an outsider looking in.

All these research tools are ways of collecting data or information.

- How was data collected in the study you are reading? Remember to record it on your summary sheet.

- With regard to the stated aim of the study you are reading and your nursing knowledge and common sense, was the most appropriate method used?

- If you do not think the method the most appropriate, why was it used? What would have been better?

- If you had used the same research tools as the author of the report would you have used them in the same way?

There are two important points that you should keep in mind when questioning the use of any research tool: it must demonstrate reliability and validity.

- **Reliability** assesses the degree to which the tool is measuring something, but good reliability does not mean that the tool is measuring what it is supposed to measure!
- **Validity** is concerned with whether the tool measures what it is supposed to measure.

There are various ways of testing that research tools are reliable and valid. If you are reading a journal article there might be only a passing mention that reliability and validity were verified, whereas research reports and theses should describe how the tools used were tested for reliability and validity.

In quantitative approaches, reliability is typically assessed by looking at the match (correlation) between two sets of scores when the same tool is used with the same group of people on two occasions. If the scores correlate, this is known as **temporal stability** (or test–retest reliability). Sometimes two forms of the same tool yield similar scores; this is referred to as alternate form reliability. Other researchers test for **internal consistency** of the research tool they plan to use by looking at how separate parts within the tool correlate; this is done by looking at the scores of the individual parts compared with the overall scores. In nursing there are times when nurses have to use their judgement about patients' behaviour or condition. The reliability of such assessments is tested by using two assessors and comparing their scores using a test of correlation, which provides an index of **interscorer/interjudge reliability**.

Validity is assessed by correlating the score with some external criterion to obtain a validity coefficient. For example, if a test was designed to assess student nurses' ability to complete a course successfully, these scores would be correlated with their course marks and a match or correlation sought. This kind of validity is called **criterion validity** (or empirical validity).

Construct validity refers to a tool that has been designed to measure some concept which forms part of a theory and that has been found to be valid in the process of theory testing.

To be satisfied of a tool's construct validity, several different ways of testing the tool and the theory are carried out.

In qualitative studies such rigid measures of validity and reliability are often not possible or even desirable. Different techniques therefore need to be considered to establish the accuracy and credibility of the tools: reliability is concerned with the accuracy and comprehensiveness of the data collected; validity focuses on the credibility of the study itself. For example, does the interpretation of the data match the recorded description of the data? Adequate documentation of the process, analysis and outcomes is thus essential if validity is to be established. The work needs to outline what is often referred to as clear decision or audit trails for the reader. It is not uncommonly claimed that such an audit is rather subjective compared to the more objective application of measurements when reviewing quantitative tools. Although this may be so to an extent, the process itself should be no less rigorous. You need to investigate how the data are used to develop pertinent themes and patterns and be given sufficient information to validate this. You also need to consider the nature of the data: are field notes (like a diary of the research) included to illuminate ideas, direct quotes from participants used to corroborate key points?

So, does the research tool used in the study actually measure what it is supposed to do (validity) in a consistent manner (reliability)? If you are reading a journal article or an abbreviated research report, you might not be in a position to make a judgement on these factors, but you do need to bear them in mind if you are thinking about implementing the findings from the study. For more details, see Gibbon (1995) or any in-depth text on research design.

There is one further point you always need to consider – bias. This is a positive or negative influence on a concept, theory or attitude and is determined by errors in the research design, e.g. in the setting and wording of the research tools, in the sample selection or in the interpretation of data.

Different research tools

Some advantages and disadvantages of research tools are considered in the following sections. Think about whether or not these are relevant to the piece of research you are reading.

Questionnaires

Advantages	Disadvantages
Can be given to several people at the same time, e.g. to a whole class.	Takes time and effort to prepare and to test for reliability and validity (see above). Might be expensive to print and reproduce.
Can be answered anonymously, therefore respondents might be more truthful.	Respondents might not be able to express their opinions or seek clarification.
Can be easier for the researcher to analyse and code responses.	Some people just do not like forms!
Respondents cannot be put off by the status of the researcher.	Respondents might complete their questionnaires casually, not bothering about their answers, so as to get the questionnaire out of the way.
Several people can answer at one time, so respondents' and researcher's time can be used more effectively.	Respondents might give the answer that they think should be given, as if they were trying to supply the correct answer in a test, especially if the researcher is in some position of power or senior to them.
	The researcher cannot ask a respondent to clarify answers.

- Were questionnaires used in the study you are reading?
- Was the questionnaire designed by the researcher?
- If so, how was its reliability and validity tested? In other words, is it reliable and does it measure what it is supposed to do?
- If you are familiar with the subject area of the research study (e.g. children in hospital), would you have asked those questions in relation to the aims of the study?
- Have important issues been missed by the questionnaire?
- Are the questions unambiguous? (If you are reading a journal the questions might not be given.)
- Are the questions suitably worded for respondents? For example, a questionnaire that asks mothers about their sick

children must be worded differently from a questionnaire to doctors treating the same group of children.

■ When were the questionnaires completed? Were the respondents tired or had they just been given bad or good news? Does the researcher give you any indication of such facts?

■ Were there any other significant factors that might have affected the answers given by the respondents?

■ Did a group of respondents complete the questionnaires together, and so perhaps talked about their answers to produce a consensus opinion rather than individual views?

I am sure you can think of several other factors that affect not only the design of questionnaires but also how they are completed; how did the researcher try to insure against these factors?

There are many articles reporting the use of questionnaires; these studies can be quantitative and/or qualitative, e.g. descriptive studies by Love (1996) and Laszlo & Strettle (1996) or the experimental study by Hicks (1996).

Interviews

Before setting out the advantages and disadvantages it is best to consider the different types of interview. In some cases it is essential that exactly the same questions are asked in exactly the same way, rather like a verbal questionnaire. This is a **structured interview**. A more flexible approach is gained from a **semi-structured interview** (e.g. Hicks et al 1996, Jerrett & Costello 1996), where the researcher has some headings or points to be covered in the interview but not a strict format. An **open ended** or **unstructured interview** is what it sounds like. Apart from setting the topic it is more like a discourse between two people. The researcher does not guide the direction or flow of the interview.

Advantages	Disadvantages
The person being interviewed, the interviewee, can seek clarification; so can the researcher.	The researcher needs to be skilled in interview techniques.
	The interviewee might not like, or be fearful of, the interviewer.
The interviewee might be able to express views and opinions more easily verbally than in writing.	The interviewee might reply as he or she thinks she should do, in order to please the researcher or to appear in a good light.

Advantages	Disadvantages
The researcher can check for misunderstandings that arise because of culture or dialect. For example, in the UK 'presently' means 'soon' or 'in a short while'; in the US, however, 'presently' means 'now' or 'at the present'.	The interviewer can bias the interview, even unwittingly, by non-verbal cues, e.g. frowning at certain information so that the interviewee does not elaborate or mention it again. The reverse can also happen.
In semi-structured or unstructured interviews, interesting lines of thought can be followed up and explored.	Interviews are time-consuming. There might be difficulties in recording the information from the interview.
The interview can provide more flexibility for the researcher and interviewee. This depends on the design of the study.	There might be difficulties in analysing and coding the information. Interviews are not anonymous.

Use your experience and knowledge to think about the situations or topics where these three types of interview would be most appropriate.

- Were interviews used in the study you are reading?
- If they were used, which type was used and do you think it was the most suitable interview schedule?
- What could have been gained or lost through using a different format for the interviews?

(Note: the interview schedule is likely to be in the appendices of the full report.)

Participant observation

Recently reported studies using participant observation will provide you with an idea of how this research tool is used.

For example, Clarke (1996) used participant observation in a secure unit and Waterman et al (1996) used participant observation as an opportunity to evaluate the introduction of case management in a rehabilitation unit for the elderly.

Advantages

The researcher is part of the situation, so might be aware of less tangible aspects such as morale, apathy, goodwill.

The researcher might be seen as having credibility by those being observed.

Disadvantages

The researcher might have difficulty in making objective observations if involved in the situation.

The researcher might have difficulty in recording observations, especially if working in a busy clinical area.

The participants involved in the observations might see the researcher as a threat or spy, affecting the accuracy of observation.

Non-participant observation

Torrance & Serginson (1996) used non-participant techniques to assess the preparation of student nurses in the measurement of arterial blood pressure. Ragneskog et al (1996) used video recording as part of a field experiment of the effect of different types of music at meal times on five patients suffering from dementia.

Advantages

As the researcher is not involved in the situation, she/he might be able to make more objective observations.

The researcher might be able to follow a plan of observation.

Disadvantages

The observer might be conspicuous, affecting what is being observed.

Two observers are often necessary to guard against observer bias.

There is a limit to the amount of time for which a researcher can observe.

It is difficult to maintain objectivity at times.

This rather long chapter has considered some of the aspects you might encounter when you read how the research study was carried out and how the information or data was collected.

I hope that some of the mystery has been taken out of this process and that your skills of enquiry and questioning have been stimulated. Now that you are aware of how the study was carried out, it is time to look at the results.

Answer to question on page 46
Level of parental knowledge: the independent variable
Infants' sleep behaviour: the dependent variable.

8

The results

Key words:
- Mean
- Median
- Mode
- Statistical significance
- Qualitative considerations
- Probability
- Chi-squared test
- *t*-test
- Standard deviation
- Ethical issues

This chapter focuses on how to set about interpreting the results of research. It initially explores the tests, terms and ways of presentation most commonly associated with quantitative research results. For some, these might appear daunting and there is not sufficient room in this book to discuss all the terms you will encounter. However, I will give you some advice that will make the results section of any quantitative research piece easier to approach. I will also define a few of the most common terms. Thus, with a little thought and a healthy dose of caution the task becomes manageable.

Although the results of qualitative research can contain some of the elements discussed in the first section of this chapter, they are normally presented in a more discursive format. Hence the second part of this chapter will alert you as to the types of issues you should be considering when analysing the results of qualitative research. Lastly, although you will probably want to explore this important topic further, key ethical implications of research will be raised.

Interpreting the results

First off, don't panic! You already know what the study is about, having read the summary and the conclusions. The results are what they say they are: findings on which the conclusions were based. However, it is important that you read the results in an informed way so that you can be sure the researcher is drawing reasonable conclusions from them. If the results show, for example, that there is a slight difference in nursing management expertise between six managers who had been in post 2 years compared with six managers who had been in post 5 years, it would be unwise (given the small sample size and the slight difference) for the researcher to conclude that length of experience affected *all* managers' expertise. In other words, to generalise from such results would be ill advised.

Second, read all titles or captions accompanying tables and figures carefully. The unclear or overwhelming will soon start to make sense if you take the time to read what it says. Do not be baffled by the figures. *Stop*, *look* and *think*. Let that be your 'highway code' to guide you safely through the results section.

Third, if you still don't understand, get help. You need to be sure that you understand the essentials of the report. This is especially important if you are thinking of implementing the findings. Sources of help can include colleagues or more detailed texts, for example Anthony (1999).

Quantitative considerations

The following terms are well worth mastering as they are used frequently. Familiarity with them will help you to understand what you are reading.

Mean

The **mean** is the arithmetic average, i.e. all the scores added together and divided by the number of scores. For example:

$$5+3+2+6+6+1+5+6+1+4+5+6+1+6+3 = 60$$

Therefore, the mean is 60/15 = 4.

Median

The **median** is the number that occurs in the middle of an ordered sequence of scores. For example, if the above scores are rearranged as:

$$1+1+1+2+3+3+4+5+5+5+6+6+6+6+6 = 60$$

the median is 5.

Mode

The **mode** is the score that occurs most frequently in a range of scores. In the above example, the score 6 occurs five times. Therefore, the mode is 6.

You can see how exactly the same scores provide a different answer depending on which arithmetical 'treatment' is used, so be careful in your reading.

> Here is a little story to help you see the relevance of each term. I had the pleasure of knowing a wonderful 82-year-old lady from Scotland. She suffered from angina, which was aggravated by the cold. Her flat faced north and was very cold in winter. But being a true Scot she was very economical. As soon as her daughter had gone to work she turned the heating off, or right down, and did not turn it up again until just before her daughter was due home! The evenings were therefore quite cosy and warm. If the temperature of the flat had been recorded every hour during the day and the *mean* (the average temperature) used as a measure of her living environment, it would probably have been above the level to worry about hypothermia. However, if readings had been taken hourly throughout the day and ranked in ascending order, the *median* (the reading in the middle of the sequence) would have given a truer picture. If the *mode* (the most frequent reading) had been used, this might have revealed a worrying but accurate picture because the temperature of the flat would have been low on six or seven occasions during the day. This information could have been clearly seen if the temperatures had been plotted on a graph.

- In your own work, when would each of these three terms be of most use to you? Make a note of your examples.

Presenting data visually

You are familiar with graphs, for example in the form of temperature charts. However, there are a number of points concerning the interpretation of graphical material that might cause you problems.

I have already highlighted the importance of reading the captions that accompany any table, graph, pie or bar chart. The titles or captions tell you about the information (data) that you are about to consider. If you are confronted with a graph or a bar chart, read the title carefully and look at the numerical ranges of both the horizontal and vertical axes.

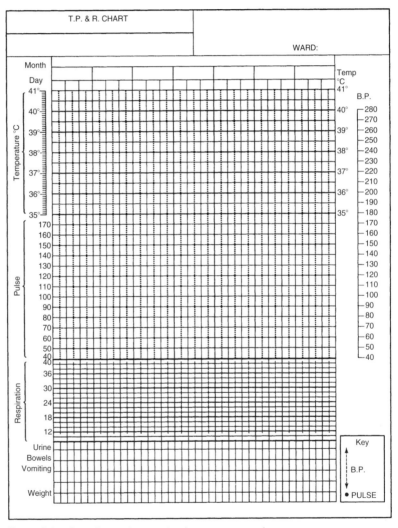

Figure 8.1   Sample graph: a patient's temperature chart.

Graphs

Figure 8.1 shows a patient's temperature chart. The caption would show the patient's name, the name of the ward or unit and whether the temperature was recorded 4-hourly, daily, and so on. The horizontal axis gives the date and time and the vertical axis is marked off in degrees Celsius.

In reality (and in Fig. 8.1) many temperature charts are three graphs one above the other, showing temperature, pulse and respiration (TPR). Each graph shares the same horizontal information (date and time) but the vertical axes for each graph are different and have different numerical ranges to reflect the nature of the recordings. For instance, in Fig. 8.1 the vertical axis for temperature ranges from 35 to 41°C; each degree is subdivided into tenths so that a patient's temperature can be recorded as, for example, 37.4°C. However, the vertical axis for pulse rate is numbered from 40 to 170 divided into tens (i.e. 40, 50, 60, etc.); each division of 10 is subdivided into fifths so that the smallest division equals two. The vertical axis for respiratory rate is numbered from 12 to 40 divided into sixes (i.e. 12, 18, 24, etc.); each division of six is subdivided into thirds so that the smallest division is again two.

Most nurses complete and/or read TPR charts accurately and with little hesitation, so remember these skills and transfer them to your appraisal of other graphs you may encounter in the report you are reading.

Figure 8.2 is taken from a study of the influence of music on the feeding and eating behaviour of patients suffering from dementia (Ragneskog et al 1996). What can you learn from a look at this graph? The graph shows the time (in minutes) five patients spent with their dinner under four conditions, three with different types of music and one control period. The graph shows at a glance that there was variation between patients and slight variation between conditions.

Pie charts

A pie chart resembles a pie divided into slices. The slices represent the size of a particular category; the larger the slice, the larger that particular category. For example, Fig. 8.3a represents the numbers of Christmas cards I usually send to different locations. The smallest slice indicates those that are sent overseas, the medium-sized slice those delivered locally and the

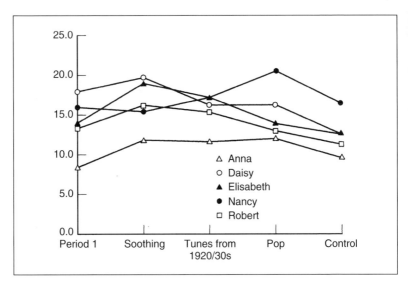

Figure 8.2   Sample graph: time spent on dinner (from Ragneskog H, Kihlgren M, Karlssonl I, Norberg A 1996 Dinner music for demented patients: analysis of video-recorded observations. Clinical Nursing Research 5:262–282. Reproduced by permission of Sage Publications, Inc.).

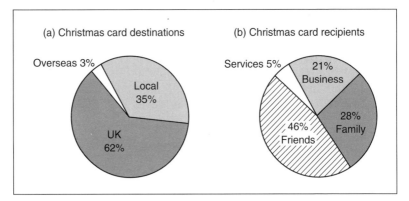

Figure 8.3   Pie charts: (a) number of cards by location, (b) number of cards sent by type of recipient.

largest slice those delivered elsewhere within the UK. I could also choose to consider how many cards were sent to businesses, service providers, family and friends, and this would produce a different pie chart (Fig. 8.3b).

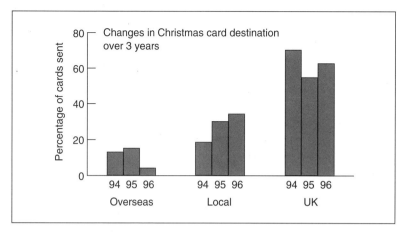

Figure 8.4   *Bar chart showing how the distribution of cards has varied over the 3 years 1994–1996.*

Bar charts

However, if I wished to see how the above distribution had changed over time it would be easier to use a bar chart (Fig. 8.4). As with graphs, look carefully at the captions and the frequency/distribution ranges along the axes.

Examine the bar chart in Fig. 8.5, taken from a journal article about how nurse teachers keep up to date (Love 1996). From this chart it is possible to see at a glance which of the activities was regarded as indispensable by the nurse teachers for keeping up to date.

■ Which activity was regarded as indispensable by nurse teachers? See page 74 for answer.

After studying these examples I hope you feel more comfortable when looking at charts, graphs and figures and realise that they are simply a way of presenting data in a more interesting way that enables you to see similarities, differences, spreads and trends at a glance. Therefore, take your time and read carefully any figures or graphs in the report you are reading.

If you still feel unhappy about interpreting data, Hicks (1994) is a clear straightforward article that covers the route from tabulated data to the presentation of that data in various graphical forms; it is well worth reading.

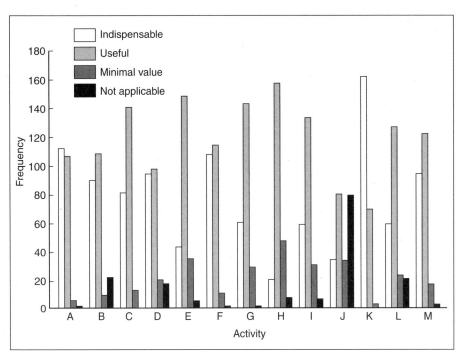

Figure 8.5   Bar chart showing how nurse teachers keep up to date (from Love C 1996 How nurse teachers keep up-to-date: their methods and practices. Nurse Education Today 16:287–295. Reproduced with permission of Churchill Livingstone).

Some terms that are frequently used in the results section of reports are now examined.

Significance (significance level, statistical significance)

We use the word 'significant' in our everyday conversations, perhaps to tell our friends about a significant point in our lives; in other words, when something memorable happened to us that might have altered the course of our lives, like getting our first job or getting married.

In research, the word 'significance' has a specific and rather precise use. It refers to **statistical significance**. When a piece of research has been carried out, especially if an experimental design was used (as in Boore (1978) and Kerr et al (1996), both discussed earlier), the researcher wants to be sure that the findings did not occur by chance or because of one or two extreme cases. In other words, how probable is it that the information given to the experimental group is low for postoperative stress or better sleep in infants is really due to the independent variable, rather than a chance happening?

Probability (*P*) is another term frequently used in reports and is closely linked to significance. Probability is a measure of whether an event is likely to occur. By convention, probability is measured from one (the event is inevitable) to zero (the event is impossible). In life, most events are somewhere in the middle. If you would like to read more, Harris (1986) provides a readable account of these issues.

Tests of significance

Having introduced these two terms, we now proceed to think about how the researcher attempts to verify that the results obtained were not due to chance. We can never be sure whether results are due to chance, but we can work out the probability that they might be due to chance; this is **statistical inference**. There are many statistical tests available, and different tests are appropriate in different conditions and situations. The choice of test is beyond the scope of this book; you will not be in a position to question whether the correct test was used. However, as you are likely to be reading published research you can assume that a panel of knowledgeable experts will have vetted the report before it was published.

Tests of significance indicate whether the difference between the observed results and those expected from the original hypothesis is likely to have been due to chance.

The **level of significance** is derived from statistical tests, the results of which are compared with statistical tables (which can be found in any statistical textbook, along with instructions to work out the test).

Chi-squared test

One of the commonly used tests of significance in many nursing research reports is the **chi-squared (χ^2) test**. This test is used on datasets that are organised into categories rather than scores.

The example below is taken from Atkinson & Sklaroff (1987). In Chapter 4 of their monograph there are several statements similar to the one below:

$$\chi^2 = 19.884, 4 \text{ df}, P < 0.001$$

where $<$ means less than and the abbreviation 'df' refers to **degrees of freedom,** which is calculated as part of the statistical test and is used to determine the level of significance. The chi-squared (χ^2) value obtained from the results of the research in the example above is compared with figures in a table of probabilities at the 4 df level.

In the context of tests of significance, probability refers to the likelihood of the experimental results differing from those expected from the original hypothesis by random chance. The nearer the value of P to zero, the smaller the likelihood that the difference between observed and expected data is due to chance and, therefore, the more significant the experimental findings.

There are accepted guidelines for assessing the significance of the difference between the observed and the expected data. When $P < 0.05$ (e.g. 0.04, 0.03, 0.02), the difference is said to be significant. For $P > 0.05$ (e.g. 0.06, 0.08, 0.1; $>$ means greater than), the difference is said to be not significant (NS). When P is much less than 0.05, the difference between the observed and expected data assumes a greater level of significance. At $P < 0.01$ and $P < 0.001$ the differences, by convention, attain significance of higher orders of magnitude. Sometimes a probability value for a chi-squared test will be followed by one, two or three asterisks, denoting probabilities of less than 0.05, 0.01 and 0.001, respectively.

t-*Test*

Another commonly used statistical test of significance is the *t*-test. The chi-squared test is a test of significance between datasets organised into categories, e.g. helpers and non-helpers, whereas the *t*-test is a significance test for the difference between two sets of scores.

Some of the research studies already mentioned have used these tests. For instance, Hicks (1996) gives the results of a *t*-test on characteristics related to the gender of researchers, whereas Clement et al (1996) used a chi-squared test to examine women's satisfaction with antenatal care and the variables that might influence satisfaction with altered frequency of visits.

Distribution

We have seen that the mean is a useful statistic. When considered with other statistics, such as the median and the mode, an idea of the **distribution** of a number of observations can be obtained. A better measure of such distribution is the **standard deviation**. This statistic is calculated from the amount by which each score differs from the mean of all scores. For example, suppose a test a group of seven student nurses (Group 1) are given marks out of 10. If the scores are 9, 1, 2, 4, 8, 5 and 6, the mean is 5 but the scores range from 9 to 1; this indicates a wide range in their knowledge. However, if another group of seven student nurses (Group 2), sitting the same test, score 6, 4, 4, 5, 5, 6 and 5, the mean is the same as Group 1 (i.e. 5) but the variation in the scores is much smaller (from 4 to 6). In this example the standard deviation for the scores differs, being higher in Group 1 where the range of scores is greater. (For further information on the calculation and interpretation of standard deviation see Reid & Boore 1987 or Couchman & Dawson 1995.) If you are reading a report that gives the result as a mean score, look at the size of the standard deviation; it could be very important. In the example above, you cannot assume that a group mean of 5, half the possible marks, demonstrates that all the students are reasonably proficient. First, *stop*, *look* and *think*. In Group 1, which had the higher standard deviation, one student scored only 1 and another 2. These scores do not indicate proficiency. Yet Group 2, with the same mean, might be considered a reasonably proficient group as only two students were 1 mark below the mean. I am sure you can think of examples in your work where a wide range of results could be very important.

Correlation

The final term discussed in this section is the **coefficient of correlation**. This is a numerical index used to indicate the degree of correspondence (match) between two sets of measurements, e.g. the degree of agreement between two nurses rating the behaviour of a hyperactive child or two nurses rating the size of varicose ulcers.

A coefficient of correlation of 1 indicates a perfect match (i.e. a one-to-one agreement); 0.9 indicates a near perfect match or correlation; 0.5 indicates only half agreement and 0.2 virtually no match or correlation; -1.0 indicates a perfect negative correlation.

There are various statistical tests used to calculate the coefficient of correlation. These are described in more detail in Reid & Boore (1987) or Couchman & Dawson (1995). Remember, the nearer to 1, the better the correlation.

Qualitative considerations

Although they might at first appear more straightforward, qualitative results can also be complex to analyse. Polit et al (2001) offer a useful five-stage framework to trigger critical questions to ask, and this is outlined below. Despite the focus being different, it is also valid to apply the same dimensions to quantitative findings:

- Stage one: are the results credible?
- Stage two: what do the results mean?
- Stage three: are the results important?
- Stage four: are the results transferable?
- Stage five: what are the implications of the results?

see
Chapter 7

Stages one and two entail analysing the results in the light of their reliability and validity as discussed in Chapter 7. Stage one requires that you make a judgement as to the credibility of the results – are they believable? What evidence is offered in their support? Given your knowledge and experience, are you persuaded by the evidence? Qualitative researchers attempt to make sense of the data as they develop and establish themes and patterns that emerge. Thus the meaning of the results – stage two – should be logically derived from this analysis. You also need to question whether you think the results are important, stage three. Did the subject warrant investigation? Was it perhaps already adequately explored by prior research? Did the findings appear rather trivial or did they provide some insightful new reflections? Qualitative studies are also 'context bound', that is, they relate to a specifically defined setting, purposeful sample, and so on. It is not, therefore, a key aim of qualitative researchers to strive for results that can necessarily be readily applied to other environments. That said, if there is no prospect of generalising from the results, they are of little value to practice. Hence the parameters of the context itself need to be considered carefully with a view to again making a judgement as to how transferable the results are (stage four).

If you have answered the questions satisfactorily in stages one to four, you then need to consider the implications of the findings – stage five. What, if any, inferences do they have for practice? Would it be beneficial for the study to be replicated in a different area of practice? Do the findings contribute in any way to existing theory? Are there aspects of the findings that would be amenable to exploration by a different research approach? These questions are by no means exhaustive but are a good starting point to commence your exploration of research findings. Use the stages as subheadings on your summary sheet as a prompt and to stimulate further thought.

Ethical issues

As with practice itself, the ethical implications of any research cannot be overlooked. It is vital to consider the moral values that underpin the process. You need to establish whether the political, legal and social obligations have been adequately fulfilled with relation to the participants by again seeking the answers to a range of questions. You need to be assured that participants were protected from any physical, psychological or indeed sociological harm or exploitation. Were they, for example, fully informed as to the nature of the study and of their rights, and did they freely give their informed consent? Were their privacy and anonymity protected? Were particularly vulnerable participants (those perhaps made vulnerable by age, disease or disability) given added protection? Was the study reviewed and/or approved by an ethics committee? These vast and complex issues are well served by an abundance of texts dedicated to the subject such as that by De Raeve (1996), and it is certainly worth consulting such sources for detailed guidance.

Summary

I hope you find these brief descriptions useful when making your way through the results section in the research report you are reading. Remember to complete your summary sheet. Remember too that at the back of this book is the Glossary, which defines the terms considered here.

 As you read more reports, you might find it helpful to compile your own dictionary of terms and questions you have added to those offered here.

Having considered the most factual part of the report, Chapter 9 moves on to consider how the researcher interprets the results in light of the aim of the study and other relevant factors.

Answer to question on page 67 is Activity K, which was reading journals.

9
The discussion and conclusion

Key words:
- Review
- Summary
- References
- Appendices

Chapters 7 and 8 introduced many terms that might have been new to you. There are no new terms in this chapter, which looks at the last parts of a research report – the discussion and conclusion. The discussion contains an analysis of the results and a **review** of the study as a whole. The conclusion is a **summary** of the whole study. When reading the discussion of your chosen report, you need to use your nursing knowledge and expertise, as well as common sense, to consider the veracity of the arguments made by the researcher.

Discussion

In this part of a research report the researcher discusses the results given in the previous section and relates them to the initial research question. The results will also be considered in relation to the work reviewed in the introduction/literature search and to any other relevant aspects (e.g. clinical applications).

Turn to your summary sheet and remind yourself about the aim of the study. If you have not yet summarised the results on to the summary sheet, do so now. Writing this summary will help you to clarify your thoughts and focus on pertinent points. Now that you have done this, there are some questions you should bear in mind as you read the discussion.

- First, has the research itself achieved its overall aim?
- Would you make the same inferences as the researcher does from what you have just read?

- How do the results of the present study support/contradict previous work?
- Is there evidence that all the results were discussed – both those that were perhaps expected, and any unanticipated findings?
- What are the limitations of the study? For example, is the study limited by sample size (consult your summary sheet)? Is the study limited by its specificity or can some findings be more widely applied (e.g. does a piece of research on weight gain in premature babies have any implications for the care of other babies)? It is important that any limitations (or weaknesses) are openly identified and discussed as these could potentially be rectified by further research.
- What implications can be drawn from the research?

Conclusion

This final part of the report summarises all that has gone before. Usually, it also points the way forward to further research and/or application of the findings.

- What has this piece of research added to the body of knowledge?
- How could or should it affect nursing care, policy, procedure or education?
- Even if the research was not carried out in your speciality, what are the implications for your area? An example of the implications of one research study being applied to a different situation can be seen in Pat Ashworth's (1980) study. This piece of research was carried out among intensive care nurses, yet the findings (about how nurses communicate or fail to communicate with patients unable to respond) have been found to be most helpful in relation to care of the elderly.
- Were the conclusions logically derived from the discussion?
- What have you learned from the research about: (i) the topic being researched; and (ii) the research process?

Now summarise the conclusion on to the summary sheet. This completes the first side of the summary sheet; the reverse side can be used to discuss how the findings could be applied in your area of nursing. (The application of research findings is discussed in Chapter 10.)

You have reached the end of the main part of the research report. The remainder of the report contains the **references**, the sources for all the material referred to during the report. If you have been reading a research report rather than a journal article there might also be a **bibliography** and **appendices**. It is likely that you will have consulted the appendices while you were look-ing at questionnaire items and/or the interview schedule.

At this point you should complete the index card you pre-pared at the start. Summarise the main points of the research report, giving just enough detail for it to make sense to you in 6 months' time. I suggest that as you complete these cards you keep a record of the subject codes you choose, as it will be dif-ficult to remember what they stand for after a few weeks or months.

With your finished report, your completed card, your notes and (I hope) your new-found confidence, this is an appropriate moment for a little reflection.

- What was your aim when you started reading the research report?
- Was it part of a course requirement or did someone else say you should read it?
- Do you understand what you have read?

If you still have doubts, consult the more detailed texts out-lined in the Further Reading section. It could be that you will need to look at the study in more depth or obtain a copy of the full report or thesis, in which case your local librarian will probably be able to help. Alternatively, a discussion with a col-league might help to clarify your ideas. Chapter 10 considers the implications of research for practice.

10

Implications for practice

Key words:
- Research-based profession
- Evidence-based practice
- Implementation

Chapters 1 and 2 focused on some of the issues concerning why a **research- and evidence-based profession** is important. Having read your piece of research with the aid of this book, you need to ask yourself:

- Has the research report any use or relevance for everyday work?

At the start of this book (p. 7) we examined the research related to pressure areas that was carried out by Doreen Norton in the 1960s and the subsequent research and clinical practice, only to find that ritual, non-research-based treatments are still being carried out. Sadly, Tross (1995), reviewing the care of wounds and pressure ulcers, reports that research-based care is still not prevalent. She concludes:

see Chapter 2

> If nurses are to be encouraged to apply research findings to the care of wounds and pressure sores, it is important for related policies and procedures to reflect such findings. Nurses must also be encouraged to consult the references provided and to review them with a critical eye, with a view to ensuring that wound care management is in line with current thinking and knowledge of the subject. (Tross 1995, p. 28)

Professor Tony Butterworth (1994) describes the long process (36 years) of a research idea with abstract theoretical beginnings that turned into an everyday practice activity. He describes psychosocial interventions with people with schizophrenia, outlining four phases and the policy matters, educational changes, service provision and various other influences on the development of the process. He concludes that research has no clear end-point, but the importance of persevering with a research idea cannot be overestimated. I would add that this applies equally to the reading and understanding of research.

Both these accounts also highlight the political, professional, clinical and, not least, personal dimensions of the research endeavour, as outlined in Chapter 2. There is certainly now evidence that the UK government is embracing the idea of research- and evidence-based practice, and this is reflected in initiatives such as clinical governance and clinical effectiveness. The National Institute of Clinical Excellence (NICE) now provides a range of excellent material on available 'best practice' for health professionals and the general public, our customers. The profession too is active in a number of ways, from publishing relevant policy documents to promoting on-going development for individual healthcare workers.

see Chapter 2

Your journey through this book should have helped you to reconsider the clinical and personal dimensions of research. So how are you going to assess the relevance of the report you have just read and address the persistent call for care to be research- and evidence-based? To a certain extent, you are already well on the way to answering this question because you have tackled a report. The following questions might help you consider how the research findings can best be applied to your nursing practice.

- Are you sure the findings are valid and reliable?
- Are there other studies or reports to support the findings?
- Are there other studies or reports to contradict the findings? You will find the references at the end of the report you have been reading useful in helping you answer the last two questions. Remember, however, that the references indicate research that was written *before* the research you are reading; you may need to conduct a literature search for more recent material.

- If you have read a summary of the research and think that it is useful to you and that the findings could be implemented, have you read the original source in order to look at all the limitations and pitfalls?

- How practical will it be to implement the findings? Look at both the costs and benefits. List them. Don't forget the hidden costs such as training time for new techniques, increased anxiety at a time of change, and so on.

■ Who would be involved in the implementation, both directly and indirectly? Don't forget issues related to the storage and disposal of equipment, porterage, unions, staff training and continuing education departments.

When you have listed all these, *stop*, *look* and *think* again.

■ Why should there be change?

■ Is the contemplated change for the better?

If, after you have answered all these questions, you still think that **implementation** of the research findings is a good idea, approach your line manager with a succinct summary of the research, including a copy of your summary sheet, the answers to the above questions and a list of advantages and disadvantages of implementation. This will make your argument more balanced from the start. Sooner or later, someone is bound to point out the contradictions, cost, implications and potential problems, so that person might as well be you. In this way you will be able to follow up with effective counterarguments.

I hope that now you feel encouraged to read research and to use the knowledge you gain in this way. I hope that you read with purpose and that, as you master the terms and concepts of the research process, you will question not only what you read but also your own practices. Such questioning is essential to the pursuit of excellence. Research is not an alien thing, it *can, does* and *must* affect everyday nursing. You do not need to undertake research yourself to examine the findings that other people present and to consider whether and how they apply to your work. In the words of Baroness McFarlane of Llandaff (1984):

> Research is thus not a luxury for the academic, but a tool for developing the quality of nursing decisions, prescriptions and action. Whether as clinicians, educators, managers or researchers we have a research responsibility; neglect of that responsibility could be classed as professional negligence.

In June 1996, the Foundation of Nursing Studies published *Putting research into practice: reflection for action*. More recently (in 2000) it published *Taking action: moving towards evidence based practice*. The Foundation's aim is to 'disseminate, use and implement proven research findings to improve patient care'. Mulhall (1996) writing about the background to the organisation states:

> Research is used when it is accessed, read and evaluated with a view to increasing knowledge and understanding. Implementation occurs when changes, based on the results of research are made in practice. These activities rely not only on the availability of relevant research, but more crucially on the critical evaluation of that knowledge.

She goes on to say how important it is that research findings are translated into the language and action of practice and that there is an opportunity to sustain change based on research findings. I hope that you will contribute to the application of research using the knowledge you have gained while reading this book.

Take heart – you are not alone. There might be a journal club in your unit or locality, or you might find there is a local research interest group. These will give you support and enable you to share interests and to form a body of research-based information.

Do you feel inspired to go on and read some more? At the very least I hope you are feeling more positive about nursing research and more ready to consider the ways in which research findings may be positively applied to improve your practice. Lathlean (1988) and indeed my work (Lanoë 1994) describes how clinical nurses have applied research findings to their work areas and altered various aspects of their practice, so it *can* be done. Now that you have made a summary of one piece of research and completed a record card, I hope you feel prepared and ready to tackle some more research reports.

Finally, the Further Reading and Reference sections provide you with books and articles that you may find useful as you continue your research reading.

References

Amos D 2001 An evaluation of staff nurse role transition. Nursing Standard 16(3):36–41

Anthony D M 1999 Nursing research: understanding advanced statistics: a guide for nursing and health care researchers. Churchill Livingstone, Edinburgh

Ashworth P 1980 Care to communicate. An investigation into the problems of communication between patients and nurses in intensive therapy units. Royal College of Nursing, London

Astbury C 1988 Stress and the nurse in the operating theatre. Royal College of Nursing, London

Atkinson F I, Sklaroff S A 1987 Acute hospital wards and the disabled patient. A survey of the experiences of patients and nurses. Royal College of Nursing, London

Ballie L 1995 Ethnography and nursing research: a critical appraisal. Nurse Researcher 3:5–21

Barrett M C, Arklie M M, Smillie C 1996 Evaluating the graduates of the Dalhousie University School of Nursing baccalaureate programme: a quantitative/qualitative responsive model. Journal of Advanced Nursing 24:1070–1076

Boore J R P 1978 Prescription for recovery. The effect of pre-operative preparation of surgical patients on post-operative stress, recovery and infection. Royal College of Nursing, London

Brazier H, Begley C M 1996 Selecting a database for literature searches in nursing: MEDLINE or CINAHL. Journal of Advanced Nursing 24:868–875

Breed S 1999 A publication guide to 40 health care journals. SB Communications Group, London

Burns N, Grove S K 2001 Practice of nursing research. W.B. Saunders, Philadelphia

Butterworth T 1994 Developing research ideas: from theory to practice. Nurse Researcher 14:78–86

Carradice A, Shankland M C, Beail N 2001 A qualitative study of the theoretical models used by UK mental health nurses to guide their assessments with family caregivers of people with dementia. International Journal of Nursing Studies 39(1):17–26

Chambers R, Boath E 2001 Clinical effectiveness and clincal governance made easy. Radcliffe Medical Press, Oxfordshire

Clarke L 1996 Participant observation in a secure unit: care, conflict and control. NTResearch 1:431–441

Clement S, Sikorski J, Wilson J, Das S, Smeeton N 1996 Women's satisfaction with traditional and reduced antenatal visit schedules. Midwifery 12:120–128

Coates V 1985 Are they being served? An investigation into the nutritional care given by nurses to acute medical patients and the influence of ward organisational patterns of care. Royal College of Nursing, London

Cortis J D, Lacey A E 1996 Measuring quality and quantity of information-giving to in-patients. Journal of Advanced Nursing 24:674–681

Couchman W, Dawson J 1995 Nursing and health-care research. A practical guide. Scutari Press, London

Department of Health 1993a Vision for the future. HMSO, London

Department of Health 1993b Report of the taskforce on the strategy for research in nursing, midwifery and health visiting, annexes 1–4. Royal College of Nursing, London

Department of Health 1994 The challenges for nursing and midwifery in the twenty first century. HMSO, London

Department of Health 1996 On research and development. HMSO, London

Department of Health 1997 The new NHS: modern, dependable. HMSO, London

Department of Health 1998 A first class service: quality in the new NHS (Health Services Circular HSC (98) 113). Department of Health, London

Department of Health and Social Security, Scottish Home and Health Department and Welsh Office 1972 Report of the committee on nursing. The Briggs Report. HMSO, London

De Raeve L (ed.) 1996 Nursing research: an ethical and legal appraisal. Baillière Tindall, London

Dubyna J, Quinn C 1996 The self-management of psychiatric medications: a pilot study. Journal of Psychiatric and Mental Health Nursing 3:297–302

East I, Robinson J 1994 Change in process: bringing about change in health care through action research. Journal of Clinical Nursing 3:57–61

Edmonstone J 1996 Strengthening cancer care: a practical approach to the empowerment of nurses. NTResearch 15:382–388

Evans K 2001 Expectations of newly qualified nurses. Nursing Standard 15(41):33–38

Faulkner A 1984 Teaching non-specialist nurses assessment skills in the aftercare of mastectomy patients. PhD Thesis, University of Manchester, Manchester

Ford P, Walsh M 1994 New rituals for old. Nursing through the looking glass. Butterworth-Heinemann, Oxford

Foundation of Nursing Studies 1996 Putting research into practice: reflection for action. Foundation of Nursing Studies, London

Foundation of Nursing Studies 2000 Taking action: moving towards evidence based practice. British Medical Association/Foundation of Nursing Studies, London

Fretwell J E 1982 Ward teaching and learning: sister and the learning environment. Royal College of Nursing, London

Fretwell J E 1985 Freedom to change. The creation of a ward learning environment. Royal College of Nursing, London

Gibbon B 1995 Validity and reliability of assessment tools. Nurse Researcher 2:48–55

Gott M 1984 Learning nursing. Royal College of Nursing, London

Grahn G, Danielson M 1996 Coping with the cancer experience. II Evaluating an education and support programme for cancer patients and their significant others. European Journal of Cancer Care 5:182–187

Granskär M, Edberg A K, Fridlund B 2001 Nursing students' experience of their first professional encounter with people having mental disorders. Journal of Psychiatric and Mental Health Nursing 8:249–256

Hallett C 1995 Understanding the phenomenological approach to research. Nurse Researcher 3:55–65

Hansebo G, Kihlgren M 2001 Carers' reflections about their video-recorded interactions with patients suffering from severe dementia. Journal of Clinical Nursing 10:737–747

Harris P 1986 Designing and reporting experiments. Open University Press, Milton Keynes

Henderson V 1987 Clinical excellence in nursing: international networking. Sigma Theta Tau International, Indianapolis

Hicks C 1994 Using tables and graphs to present research findings. Nurse Researcher 2:54–74

Hicks C 1996 The potential impact of gender stereotypes for nursing research. Journal of Advanced Nursing 24:1006–1013

Hicks C, Hennessy D, Cooper J, Barwell F 1996 Investigating attitudes to research in primary health care teams. Journal of Advanced Nursing 24:1033–1041

Hsu H-Y, Gallinagh R 2001 The relationships between health beliefs and utilization of free health examinations in older people living in a community setting in Taiwan. Journal of Advanced Nursing 35:864–873

Jerrett M D, Costello E A 1996 Gaining control: parents' experiences of accommodating children's asthma. Clinical Nursing Research 5:294–308

Kerr S M, Jowett S A, Smith L N 1996 Preventing sleep problems in infants: a randomized controlled trial. Journal of Advanced Nursing 24:938–942

Kirkevold M, Berg K, Saltvold S 1996 Patterns of recovery among Norwegian heart surgery patients. Journal of Advanced Nursing 24:943–951

Lanoë N R 1994 Research awareness in practice: a case study approach. MSc Thesis, University of Surrey, Guildford

Laszlo H, Strettle R 1996 Midwives' motivation for continuing education. Nurse Education Today 16:363–367

Lathlean J 1988 Research in action: developing the role of the ward sister. Kings Fund Centre, London

Love C 1996 How nurse teachers keep up-to-date: their methods and practices. Nurse Education Today 16:287–295

McFarlane of Llandaff 1984 The future. In: Cormack D F (ed.) The research process in nursing. Blackwell Scientific Publications, Oxford

Mead D 1996 Teaching nursing and midwifery research. In: De Raeve L (ed.) Nursing research: an ethical and legal appraisal Baillière Tindall, London, pp. 160–182

Moon J-S, Cho K-S 2001 The effects of handholding on anxiety in cataract surgery patients under local anaesthesia. Journal of Advanced Nursing 35:407–415

Moorbath P 1995 Libraries for nursing/RCN survey on access to libraries for qualified nurses. Libraries for Nursing Bulletin 15:13–31

Moores Y 1996 The research agenda: change, challenge, opportunity. NTResearch 1:330–331

Mulhall A 1996 Background to putting research into practice: reflection for action. Foundation of Nursing Studies, London

Mutasa H C F 2001 Risk factors associated with noncompliance with method substitution therapy (MST) and relapse among chronic opiate users in an outer London community. Journal of Advanced Nursing 35:97–107

Newton C A 1995 Action research: application in practice. Nurse Researcher 2:60–71

Norton D, McLaren R, Exton-Smith N 1962 An investigation of geriatric nursing problems in hospital. Churchill Livingstone, Edinburgh

Ogier M E 1982 An ideal sister? Royal College of Nursing, London

Polit D F, Beck C T, Hungler B P 2001 Essentials of nursing research: methods, appraisal, and utilization. Lippincott, Philadelphia

Powell D 1982 Learning to relate? Royal College of Nursing, London

Ragneskog H, Kihlgren M, Karlsson I, Norberg A 1996 Dinner music for demented patients: analysis of video-recorded observations. Clinical Nursing Research 5:262–282

Reid N G, Boore J R P 1987 Research methods and statistics in health care. Edward Arnold, London

Royal College of Nursing 2001 Pressure ulcer risk assessment and prevention. RCN, London

Runciman P, Currie C T, Nicol M, McKay V 1996 Discharge of elderly people from an accident and emergency department: evaluation of health visitor follow-up. Journal of Advanced Nursing 24:711–718

Russell C K, Gregory D M 1993 Issues for consideration when choosing a qualitative data management system. Journal of Advanced Nursing 18:1806–1816

Savage J 1995 Nursing intimacy: an ethnographic approach to nurse–patient interaction. Scutari Press, London

Sleep J 1988 Reported in: Advances in Midwifery Research. Senior Nurse 8:5

Spouse J 1990 An ethos for learning. Scutari Press, London

Stodulski A H 1995 Royal College of Nursing study of UK nursing journals. RCN Library Information Services, London

Stonehouse J, Butcher J 1996 Phlebitis associated with peripheral cannulae. Professional Nurse 12:51–54

Torrance C, Serginson E 1996 An observational study of student nurses' measurement of arterial blood pressure by sphygmomanometry and auscultation. Nurse Education Today 16:282–286

Tross G 1995 Raising the issues. Journal of Community Nursing 9:26–28

Twomey M 1987 Coping with mastectomy. Senior Nurse 7:10–11

United Kingdom Central Council for Nursing, Midwifery and Health Visiting 1992 Code of professional conduct for the nurse, midwife and health visitor, 3rd edn. UKCC, London

United Kingdom Central Council for Nursing, Midwifery and Health Visiting 2001a Professional self-regulation and clinical governance. UKCC, London

United Kingdom Central Council for Nursing, Midwifery and Health Visiting 2001b The PREP handbook. UKCC, London

Ward R 2001 Internet skills for nurses. Nursing Standard 15(21):47–53

Waterman H 1995 Distinguishing between 'traditional' and action research. Nurse Researcher 2:15–23

Waterman H, Waters K, Awenat Y 1996 The introduction of case management on a rehabilitation floor. Journal of Advanced Nursing 24:960–967

West B J 1992 Action research and standards of care. The prevention and treatment of pressure sores in the elderly. Scottish Health Bulletin 6:356–361

Further reading

Where to start

One encouraging change that has occurred since the first edition of this book was published in 1989 is the sheer volume of quality, complementary and accessible texts that are now available. Those mentioned below are therefore merely examples that you might find useful rather than in any way a definitive guide. Do not be constrained by this but use it perhaps to commence your voyage of exploration.

Powers B A, Knapp T R 1995 A dictionary of nursing theory and research. Sage Publications, London. A dictionary, but some of the definitions amount to explanations of several pages. A really useful book to have if you are a novice to research, and indeed on occasion if you are not!

Clamp C G, Gough S 1999 Resources for nursing research: an annotated bibliography. Corwin Press, London. This brings together literature relating to all aspects of research. It has breadth rather than depth and thus is a useful resource to dip into.

Texts about research

Buckeldee J, McMahon R 1994 The research experience in nursing. Chapman & Hall, London. Includes chapters on defining the research question, choosing a methodology, piloting a study, conducting interviews and making sense of data.

Cormack D F S (ed.) 2000 The research process in nursing, 3rd edn. Blackwell Scientific Publications, Oxford. Many students find this text helpful.

Lobiondo-Wood G, Haber J 1998 Nursing research: methods, critical appraisal and utilization, 4th edn. Mosby, St Louis. Another useful overview for the enquiring novice growing in experience and confidence.

Langford R W 2001 Navigating the maze of nursing research: an interactive learning adventure. Mosby, St Louis. I reviewed this American text for the UK market and enjoyed its friendly and fun style of presentation.

Qualitative research

Morse J M 1995 Nursing research: the application of qualitative approaches. Croom Helm (reprinted by Chapman & Hall), London. A very readable applied overview.

Morse J M (ed.) 1992 Qualitative research methods for health professionals. Sage Publications, London. Contains chapters on topics such as phenomenology, ethnomethodology, grounded theory, etc.

Bannister P, Burman E, Parker I et al 1994 Qualitative methods in psychology: a research guide. Open University Press, Buckingham. A more advanced text on qualitative research methods.

Crotty M 1996 Phenomenology and nursing research. Churchill Livingstone, Edinburgh. A more detailed review of this specific methodology.

Ethics and research

De Raeve L (ed.) 1996 Nursing research: an ethical and legal appraisal. Baillière Tindall, London. Louise De Raeve has collected contributions from 12 authors on various topics related to ethics and nursing; you will find them interesting and thoroughly grounded in nursing. An essential read for any nurse.

See also **Clamp & Gough** 1999 (details on p. 89); **Tarling M, Crofts L K** 2002 The essential researcher's handbook. Baillière Tindall, London; **Crookes P, Davies S** 2002 Research into practice. Baillière Tindall, London.

Statistics

Rowntree D 1988 Statistics without tears: a primer for non-mathematicians. Penguin, Middlesex. This readily accessible book is ideal for those new to this subject. It is described as a tutorial in print and can be used as such. However, it can also be used like a dictionary. It won't work miracles: although it promises statistics without tears, this does not mean that an understanding comes without effort!

Anthony D M 1999 Understanding advanced statistics: a guide for nursing and health care researchers. Churchill Livingstone, Edinburgh. As implied by the title, this is a more detailed and applied text, useful for the more competent, or indeed as a reference resource.

Journals

If you have been asked to look at research on a particular topic, then a computer search will provide information quickly. However, there is a lag of about 6 months before references are included on the database, so for the most recent work you will need to turn to journals. Since the first edition of this book was published there has been a proliferation of nursing journals. Ann Stodulski (formerly Librarian at the Royal College of Nursing) compiled a report on UK nursing journals entitled *Royal College of Nursing study of UK nursing journals (1995)*. Should you want your own copy it is obtainable from the RCN Library Information Services, price £15. The journals listed below were identified as featuring research reports on a regular basis:

- *Journal of Advanced Nursing*
- *Intensive and Critical Care Nursing*
- *International Journal of Nursing Studies*
- *Journal of Psychiatric and Mental Health Nursing*
- *Midwifery*
- *Nurse Education Today*
- *Nurse Researcher.*

You might find help with understanding the research process by looking at specific issues of *Nurse Researcher*, a journal of research methodology published quarterly. It is aimed at pre- and post-registration students and nurses in practice and education, with papers on research methods related to useful examples of clinical practice. Each issue has a specific theme, e.g. sampling, interviewing, observational studies, action research, ethnography and phenomenology. Volume 1, number 1 was published in September 1993 and, over the years, a useful collection of papers and ideas has accrued.

Even since Ann Stodulski produced her report in 1995, other journals have appeared and, with the push for a evidence-based practice, more and more journals are increasing their research content. For instance, *NTResearch* is a bimonthly journal that aims to publish research on nursing topics and themes; unfortunately, the references are in very small print at present. Each month during 1995, the *Journal of Community Nursing* included an article on the research process.

There are other nursing research journals that are produced outside the UK. I have used at least two references from *Clinical Nursing Research*, an international journal produced in Canada that publishes refereed articles that focus on clinical practice.

Actual research reports

The Royal College of Nursing used to publish completed doctoral and masters theses in abbreviated form, which were accessible and easily readable. The last one was published in 1994.

In 1974, the Steinberg Collection of theses and dissertations, either by nurses or on topics related to nursing in the UK, was set up and is housed in the Royal College of Nursing. In 1995, there were 724 items from 128 universities in the collection. You can obtain these on loan only through university libraries or from the British Library Document Supply Centre. A catalogue is available. However, might I suggest that this is not your first line of enquiry. Most researchers will have published journal articles or an abbreviated form of the work in the RCN Research Series. You might need to refer to the original work if you are unclear about the results or methodology and wish to clarify these before thinking about implementing the findings.

Online resources and websites

see
Chapter 3

Another major change in relation to the availability of information is the internet. As noted in Chapter 3, homepages, online databases and so on are now a valuable resource for the practitioner. Specific internet address links (uniform resource locators or URLs) have not been given in this book because these tend to change quite frequently. The most useful are easily accessible through any of the popular search engines, or current URLs can be found in recent journal articles.

Once you have identified information of interest it will of course have to be evaluated just as you would evaluate information from books or journals. The pointers in this book apply equally to electronic sources as to hard copy. However, given the lack of professional 'policing' on the internet and the fact that the quality of web-based resources can vary greatly, it is important to proceed with caution. Ward (2001) outlines some useful guides that can be applied when evaluating online resources.

see
Chapter 4

If you intend to use information from online sources this will also need referencing. In addition to the standard details demanded (as outlined in Chapter 4) you will also need to make a note of the title of the web page, medium or type of resource, location, date of access, etc. Diligently follow any 'house' rules provided, as with a standard referencing system. Remember that the overriding rule of thumb for any reference is that it should be identifiable and accessible by others.

Chapter 3

Glossary

Abstract (page 16) (at the beginning of a research report or thesis) A summary of why the study was done and the main results.

Abstracting journal (page 19) A publication that summarises published material in a particular subject area.

Action research (page 42) A method of undertaking social research that incorporates the researcher's involvement as a direct and deliberate part of the research, i.e. the researcher acts as a change agent.

Appendices (page 77) The purpose of the appendices is to expand on information that was mentioned only briefly in the report, e.g. instructions to subjects, questionnaires, interview or observation schedules.

Bias (page 54) Any tendency for results to differ from the true value in some consistent way. This could be due to experimenter bias (lack of objectivity), sample bias (non-random sample) or statistical bias (within the statistical analysis chosen).

Bibliographic software (page 22) A commercial computer disk that is supplied with templates that allow the storage, cross-referencing and retrieval of references, abstracts and notes. Some disks will also format references into various styles for printing.

Bibliography (page 77) List of material that has been read and which informs the study but that has not been referred to within the text.

British Nursing Index (BNI) (page 18) A database incorporating the RCN *Nursing Bibliography*, RCN Nurse ROM and the Nursing and Midwifery Index. Includes over 220 health-related journals, with 9000 references being added each year. Produced for the internet, on CD-ROM and in printed form.

CD-ROM (page 15) A computer disk imprinted with information that can be accessed and read but information cannot be added.

Chi-squared (χ^2) (page 69) A statistical test based on the frequencies with which events occur. It demonstrates the expected distribution of the sum of squares for scores according to the normal (bell-shaped) curve .

CINAHL (page 16) Cumulative Index to Nursing and Allied Health Literature, a CD-ROM.

Coefficient of correlation (page 71) A numerical index used to indicate the degree of correspondence (match) between two sets of measurements.

Construct validity (page 53) Refers to whether the research tool forms an accurate assessment of the theoretical construct that it is supposed to measure. Does it accurately reflect the theory underlying the idea?

Control group (page 45) A group of participants/subjects (people or things) who, in the course of an experimental research project, do not experience the factor under consideration, so that a comparison can be made with the effects produced on the **experimental group**.

Criterion validity (page 53) When validity is assessed by measuring it against some external criterion, e.g. comparing nursing exam results with IQ scores.

Cross-sectional study (page 44) Involves the comparison of two or more groups at one point in time.

Data (page 15) 'Raw' or unprocessed information or facts from which others may be inferred.

Database (page 15) A source that contains information or facts.

Degrees of freedom (df) (page 70) Associated with sampling distribution and is calculated as part of a test of significance.

Dependent variable (in experimental research) (page 45) The aspect being studied to see whether the experimental factor, the **independent variable**, has had any effect.

Descriptive research (page 42) Research that aims to provide a knowledge base when little is known of a phenomenon or to clarify a situation or describe participant characteristics, e.g. surveys, case studies, grounded theory.

Distribution (page 71) The relative frequencies with which scores of different size occur. See **standard deviation**.

Ethics (page 41) The philosophical study of the moral value of human conduct and of the rules and principles that ought to govern it.

Ethnography (page 48) A qualitative research approach developed by anthropologists with the purpose of describing an aspect of culture, but is also aimed at learning about the culture or factor being studied.

Evidence-based practice (page 2) Clinical practice that is underpinned by quality evidence (rather than being based on tradition, custom or practice) so as to deliver the best possible care, nursing or otherwise.

Experimental group (page 45) A group of participants/subjects (people or things) who, in the course of an experimental research project, are caused to experience the factor under consideration.

Experimental research (page 42) Research that tests a hypothesis by means of controlled manipulation of variables.

Hardware (page 22) Equipment used in a computer system such as the central processing unit, peripheral devices and memory.

Hypothesis (page 38) A statement based on knowledge or information that has yet to be proved or disproved, supported or rejected.

Implementation (page 81) Carrying out or putting into action.

Independent variable (in experimental research) (page 45) The experimental factor that is deliberately manipulated; it is given to the experimental group and not the control group.

Information technology (page 15) The technology of the production, storage and communication of information using computers and microelectronics.

Internal consistency (page 53) A measure of reliability in which separate items in a test are correlated with the total scores for the test.

Interscorer/interjudge reliability (page 53) A test of reliability when subjective judgements are involved in an assessment situation. The scores from two independent raters are correlated to look for agreement between them.

Interviews (page 44) Formal discussions between two people, usually for a specific purpose.

Key words (page 13) Significant words used to describe the content of a document, chapter or idea.

Level of significance (page 69) The probability of rejecting the null hypothesis when the result of statistical tests of significance is, for example, 0.05 or lower (5% level of significance). See **statistical significance** and **statistical inference**.

Literature review (page 31) A brief résumé of previous and related work.

Longitudinal study (page 44) A group of people are studied over time in order to follow any development or change in a dependent variable.

Mean (page 62) The arithmetic average.

Median (page 62) The number that occurs in the middle of an ordered sequence of scores.

MEDLINE (page 16) Computer database that covers over 4000 journals and 11 million references, mainly from the US.

Method/methodology (page 40) The way in which the researcher has tried to fulfil the aim of the study. Methodology includes such aspects as the type of research employed, sample size and selection, research tools used and ways of collecting and analysing data.

Mode (page 63) The score that occurs most frequently in a set of scores.

Non-participant observation (page 52) When the observer is not part of the situation being observed.

Null hypothesis (page 39) This states that there will be no difference in the dependent variable between the control and experimental groups (i.e. that the experiment will not work). The null hypothesis will be discarded if the experimental hypothesis is supported.

Observations (page 44) See **participant observation** and **non-participant observation**.

Participant observation (page 52) When an observer takes part in a situation that is being observed.

Participants (page 32) Any individuals who are willingly involved in the research study, who freely consent to be part of the process of providing the researcher with relevant information through observation, questioning, etc. Formerly known as subjects.

Phenomenology (page 48) A method of inquiry that looks at what life experiences are like for people.

Pilot study (page 52) A preliminary study carried out to test the proposed method and research tools for the main study.

Population (page 49) The total number of people or things that could be treated as participants/subjects in a research project.

Probability (P) (page 69) The likelihood of an event occurring by chance, rather than being caused by the experimental variables. P is expressed numerically on a scale from 0 to 1.

Qualitative research (page 31) Research that paints a picture in words and aims to identify concepts and common themes.

Quantitative research (page 31) Research in which the data are numerical and seeks to test hypotheses by statistical analysis of the data.

Questionnaires (page 44) Written lists of questions. They come in various forms from the open-ended, such as 'what do you think about…', to the forced choice, where the respondents can only answer 'yes' or 'no' to the question.

Random sampling (page 49) The systematic selection of a sample to ensure that all members of a population stand an equal chance of being selected.

Randomised controlled trial (page 46) An experimental design characterised by the manipulation of the **independent variable**. Participants are randomly assigned to the conditions (i.e. **experimental group** or **control group**) and all other factors are controlled.

References (page 22) The list of books and journals that have been cited in the text.

Reliability (of a test) (page 53) Whether the same test will give the same results when used under the same conditions on different occasions.

Research-based profession (page 2) When nursing uses research methods and research findings to assess, plan, implement and evaluate nursing care. Research informs problem-solving, decision-making and all aspects of nursing.

Research design (page 41) The selection of the most appropriate method of inquiry that will answer the research questions and aim of the study. Can be qualitative or quantitative, descriptive, experimental or action research.

Research tools (page 41) Tools used to carry out research, e.g. questionnaires, audio and video recording, interview schedules, observations (either behavioural or physiological, participant or non-participant).

Sample (page 41) A selection of people or things from the possible **population**.

Semi-structured interview (page 56) An interview in which there is some framework to the discussion, although this is in the form of subject headings rather than precise questions.

Software (page 22) Computer programs as opposed to the computer itself.

Standard deviation (page 71) A measure of distribution, calculated from the amount by which each score differs from the mean of all scores.

Statistical inference (page 69) Drawn from the testing of data for level of significance. In other words, whether it is likely that the results obtained were due to chance or due to the independent variable. See **level of significance** and **statistical significance**.

Statistical significance (page 68) A conclusion that the results achieved have little probability of occurring by chance alone. If the result is statistically significant, e.g. below the 0.05 level (i.e. 1 in 20), then we can be fairly confident that something other than chance produced the result.

Structured interview (page 56) An interview in which the discussion is carried out in a very precise manner, addressing the same issues in the same way for all participants, rather like a verbal questionnaire.

Synonym (page 13) A word that means the same or nearly the same as another word.

Temporal stability (page 53) When a research tool has been tested for reliability using the test–retest method. In other words, the tool is given to the same group of people on two occasions and the scores on the first occasion correlate with the scores on the second occasion.

Tests of significance (page 69) Tests indicating whether the difference between the observed results and those expected from the original hypothesis are likely to be due to chance.

t-test (page 70) A test of significance that is distribution dependent.

Unstructured or open interview (page 56) An interview in which there is no format or framework from which to carry out the interview; only the subject of the discussion is stated.

Validity (page 53) (of a test) Whether or not the test measures what it is supposed to measure.

Variable (page 45) An attribute, quality or characteristic that can be varied, observed and measured. See **dependent variable** and **independent variable**.

Website (page 18) pages of graphically presented material on the internet.